The
Stem Cell
REVOLUTION

Mark Berman, MD; Elliot Lander, MD

authorHOUSE®

AuthorHouse™
1663 Liberty Drive
Bloomington, IN 47403
www.authorhouse.com
Phone: 1 (800) 839-8640

Published by AuthorHouse 10/09/2015

ISBN: 978-1-5049-2001-8 (sc)
ISBN: 978-1-5049-2000-1 (hc)
ISBN: 978-1-5049-2002-5 (e)

Library of Congress Control Number: 2015910573

Print information available on the last page.

ABOUT THE COVER

In 1508, Michaelangelo Buonarroti painted this image of the creation of Adam on the ceiling of the Sistine Chapel. He not only displayed artistic genius but also possessed much knowledge as an anatomist. We now know that Michaelangelo secretly practiced his passion for anatomy at a time when the Church decreed dissection of cadavers punishable by death. He risked his career and his life in his pursuit of anatomic truth and he left us a hidden message in his juxtaposition of God with a cross section of the human brain. The image demonstrates the frontal lobe, the sulci, the hypothalamus, the brainstem, the optic chiasm, and many of the anatomic structures we first learned about in our medical school neuro-anatomy courses. American Neurologist Frank Meshberger first noted this stunning depiction of God as the supreme intelligence during an artistic epiphany while staring at the chapel ceiling nearly 500 years after it was painted. One starts to ponder what other sublime wonders lay hidden in full view. The serendipitous discovery of millions of healing stem cells programed for human repair sitting in plain view just under our skin might just be one of those wonders. We now stand at the inception of a new field of medical science. Call it regenerative science or call it "the hand of God," either way, it compels the question: what is one willing to risk for the pursuit of knowledge and truth?

Elliot Lander MD

TABLE OF CONTENTS

FOREWORD

In his bestselling 2007 book *The Black Swan*, author Nassim Taleb describes uncertainty and randomness and how we routinely underestimate huge deviations from what we expect to happen. Taleb's book weaves together philosophy, math, history, and business to explain the huge impact of highly unpredictable and improbable "Black Swan" events.

The serendipitous finding of high numbers of regenerative stem cells in the fatty tissue just under our skin – and the simple use of minor, low-risk surgical procedures and FDA-approved enzymes to release and deploy them to help heal our body's damaged tissues – combine to produce a truly extraordinary "Black Swan" event wherein every patient can be his or her own bio-factory for regenerative medicine. One might call it "Regenaceutical" as opposed to "Pharmaceutical."

How all this will impact the medical world of cell therapy, the academic world of pathways and patents, and the pharmaceutical industry, is still unclear – but the effects have already started and taken hold. That's why we call our project the "Stem Cell Revolution®."

Mark Berman, MD and Elliot Lander, MD
Founders: California Stem Cell Treatment Center and the Cell Surgical Network

PROLOGUE

We have entered the rapidly evolving stem cell age. The media saturates us with stories, hype and promises about stem cell wonders and cures. As clinicians, we witnessed the initial achievements in cell therapy unlocking the potential for actual organ repair and replacement. While academia and industry may eventually provide pharmaceutical "stem cells in a bottle," there already exists an alternative clinical industry of stem cell treatment clinics offering cell therapies derived from adult tissues – particularly adipose tissue. These centers offer patients treatment options that they cannot obtain in many traditional doctors' offices or large trials. In the US, same day surgical procedures permit physicians to transfer tissues rich in stem cells to damaged areas of the body providing patients access to regenerative therapies now. Same day surgical procedures that maintain sterility without risk of disease transmission support the very mission of the current FDA tissue handling rules. Thus, stem cells found in autologous fat, extracted through a safe and near painless procedure afford such clinics the opportunity to help countless patients now.

In 2008, colleagues in Asia provided Dr. Mark Berman, an internationally recognized expert on fat grafting procedures, an improved way to harvest and process fat for grafting. Further, they had developed a method to procure stromal vascular fraction (SVF – rich in mesenchymal stem cells) from fat. Once safe enzyme materials were available, we modified the technique to produce a closed sterile surgical method for producing SVF. We quickly realized that we had valuable technology at our disposal but that we would have to use it judiciously. From the start, we created the California Stem Cell Treatment Center®, a multispecialty team necessary for treating conditions beyond our scope of practice such orthopedic, cardio/pulmonary, urologic and other diseases. We set up safety studies for the investigational use of SVF and obtained Institutional Review Board (IRB) approval for them. We built an educational website www. stemcellrevolution.com that explains the nature of this patient funded research. We coined the term "*cell surgery*" since our surgical procedure has no laboratory component thus distinguishing ourselves from the pharmaceutical model. We have now performed over 2000 cases demonstrating extraordinary safety and no serious adverse effects related to SVF deployment. We have seen astonishing results in tissue healing, autoimmune and neurodegenerative disease mitigation, arthritis mitigation and treatment of crippling back pain. The uses and various methods of deploying SVF are continually growing.

Understanding the importance and necessity of teaching our technology to other interested physicians, we formed the Cell Surgical Network®(CSN) in 2012 and started training select physicians in our regenerative medicine techniques. CSN® now includes 79 centers around the world. All Network physicians are performing cell surgery using identical methods and protocols and all are collecting safety and outcomes data in our online database. Our safety study for the first 1000 patients is in manuscript form.

Considered a disruptive technology, point of care production and deployment of SVF allows surgeons to tap the human storehouse of healing cells, making them "bio-available" for disease mitigation. The Cell Surgical Network® mission is to accelerate the quality of regenerative medicine and have safe and cost effective cell based therapies available soon to everyone in the world. A vision we get closer to achieving every day.

Elliot Lander MD and Mark Berman MD

Chapter 1 ————

THE SCIENCE OF STEM CELLS

Stem cell: an unspecialized cell that can differentiate (i.e. change into) a specific specialized cell; also has the capability to replicate.

The mention of stem cells raises tremendous controversy, such that the American public tends to presume two things: 1) That the cells in question are embryonic cells, harvested from the tissue of aborted fetuses, or dead fetuses created and altered in a laboratory for scientific purposes, and 2) That actual operations using stem cells derived from human tissue will be a phenomenon of the distant future – they won't be available here in the United States for at least another decade. Yet here at the California Stem Cell Treatment Center, our patients have been receiving "stem-cell" injections since December of 2010. If conventional thinking places stem cells squarely in the future, how is it possible for us to offer leading-edge treatment right now? And is this even legal?

For starters, the cells that our team works with are non-embryonic cells; CSCTC uses strictly adult (not fetal) tissue and autologous cells, meaning the cells are taken from the person that receives them – donor and recipient are one and the same. Embryonic cells are hailed in the media for their pluripotent property, meaning they can differentiate into any type of cell in the body. However, embryonic cells don't relate well to adult tissue; they want to grow into a fetus, which is abnormally rapid growth in any context other than a pregnancy, resulting in the formation of teratomas which is a type of uncontrolled neoplastic (cancerous) growth. Such tumor formation has been clinically documented and has severely limited the clinical use of embryonic stem cells which is problematic since most of the basic science stem cell work done in the past 15 years has been using these embryonic cells. The adult cells that we use at CSCTC are not pluripotent, but they are plenty potent for regenerative healing. These adult stem cells (ASCs) derived from fat have been documented to be capable of forming nearly every type of tissue in the human body except placental tissue. We have proof that fat derived stem cells can form nerve tissue and other complex organs. (See addendum- History of Adipose Derived SVF).

Learn to love your body fat: It's loaded with mesenchymal stem cells, a.k.a. multipotent stromal cells, or MSCs, that can differentiate into a variety of cell types. These same cells may also be isolated from several other sources in the body, including bone marrow and the umbilical cord (cord blood cells are adult cells, not embryonic ones). For millennia, the lifeline joining mother and infant was discarded after birth; in recent years, however, growing scientific awareness that the umbilical cord is a rich reserve of stem cells has spurred the development of technology enabling parents to choose the option of having their cord blood preserved and cryobanked (deep frozen at -190°C) for their own and their children's future medical use. However, the focus on the cryopreservation of cells has been to bank HSC's also known as hematopoetic stem cells, which are a type of stem cell that is especially intended to form blood products and can be useful in patients that have blood line tumors like leukemia and need therapies that destroy the persons own blood and immune cells which then need to be repopulated with HSC's. There are a very small number of MSC's in umbilical cord but this is a poor source compared to fat.

Bone marrow MSCs have been used for a number of years, particularly for a variety of orthopedic conditions; however, they are found in relatively low numbers, and require FDA approved laboratory growth (using GMP also known as "good manufacturing practices") to ensure adequate amounts for regenerative purposes. Also, with chronic illness and advanced age the bone marrow is suppressed, and this negatively impacts the quality and quantity of the cells. As cancer patients who have undergone harvesting of their bone marrow appreciate, the removal process is difficult, painful, and invasive. As noted above, the

MSCs used at our practice are adipose-derived cells, meaning they are harvested from the patient's own fatty tissue. It turns out that fat has 2,500 times the number of MSCs as bone marrow; the cells simply lie dormant in the collagen matrix of the fat, but can be made readily available for release and bio-available to our damaged tissue for repair purposes. Scientists abbreviate the term adipose-derived stem cells as ASC, to distinguish them from bone-marrow-derived stem cells, or BSC. While different camps will try to argue that bone marrow cells have advantages over fat-derived cells, studies show that the cells derived from fat are equal – if not superior – in regenerative potency to the stem cells derived from bone marrow.

At CSCTC we employ a "mini-liposuction" technique to remove the fatty tissue. Liposuction has been the single most popular cosmetic procedure in the United States for several years now. Of course, with basic liposuction the goal is to remove unwanted fat that the patient can't otherwise lose by normal diet and exercise. Amazingly, while fat frequently finds use in transplantation for facial rejuvenation, breast augmentation, buttock augmentation, and a variety of "defect" repairs, it is otherwise largely discarded. Today, we know that there are 500,000 to 1 million stem cells in each milliliter of fat – yet during routine cosmetic procedures, surgeons were discarding what amounted to billions of these incredibly important regenerative cells. In most cases, the MSC-rich adipose tissue continues to be discarded. Most liposuction procedures require some type of sedation in addition to local anesthesia; however, at CSCTC we've developed a very rapid and simple technique for harvesting fat using only local anesthesia. It's over in about 15 minutes. Even doctors that perform liposuction that have had the procedure done on themselves find it surprisingly pain-free and simple. "It's like going to the dentist," they say (plus, it's usually a lot less painful).

The cosmetic surgeon and the urologist may seem like the premise for a "two doctors walk into a bar" joke. But believe it or not, it took exactly this medical odd couple to start a stem cell practice despite the mainstream media and medical community's insistence that stem cells are the stuff of theory, not practice – and to make this therapy available today to people who need it.

As a top cosmetic surgeon in Beverly Hills renowned for face lifts, Mark kept current with scientific studies of adipose tissue all over the world, fascinated by what was becoming increasingly evident: that "the magic of fat" went far beyond the cosmetic surgeon's gift for rejuvenating aging faces. ASC's healing potential may be easily, safely, and efficiently harvested and repurposed for therapeutic purposes including arthritis and orthopedic injury. Mark felt a professional duty to deploy SVF to help patients with more than just aesthetic medical issues. But, as a cosmetic surgeon, he would've been beyond his scope of practice if he were to start treating joint conditions. So he convinced a leading Westside orthopedic surgeon, Dr. Thomas Grogan, to consider treating patients with him. After discussing the possibilities, Grogan agreed to evaluate patients sent by Mark. Pretty soon, patients were asking Mark to address their issues with aging joints instead of aging faces.

Our original concepts were developed based on a casual conversation…"I remember when Mark returned from Japan and was sitting with me talking about how using stem cells for cosmetics was actually a waste of valuable cells when one considers the tremendous therapeutic potential of these cells. It was one of those epiphany moments and I told Mark he was right and not only was he right, but that we were going to do just that. But we both understood that we had to do it correctly. We did not want to get painted with the same broad strokes as those clinics that offered cell therapy but without rigorous protocols, data collection, and standardization of procedures. Mark and I decided to study the investigational use of stem cells found in stromal vascular fraction and offer it to our patients ethically and safely. We understood that we had to charge our patients but we set fair rates and called it patient funded research. After all, who else would fund such a project? Government and private industry had no industry in funding the study of a person's fat derived stem cells- a personal biologic that was not patentable or capable of being manufactured for commercial purposes."

Elliot as a urologist, quickly began thinking about treating so many urologic degenerative disease, such as erectile dysfunction which afflicts some 65 million Americans. The possibilities were unlimited: if this could be done as a surgical procedure rather than a laboratory based product application, then cell therapy could be made readily available to patients everywhere in the world today without an expensive laboratory or inaccessible university research program.

A cosmetic surgeon... a urologist... well, who else is going to undertake this work? There is no special residency or training for stem cell therapy. But if you're a surgeon, and someone arrives from Japan to hand you a new recipe with tremendous healing potential, aren't you obligated to do something with it, to help people? We think so. We're all physicians before we differentiate into specialists. Eager to help patients struggling with medical issues that were more than just cosmetic, and anticipating demand for this exciting new therapy, Mark crossed over into therapeutic practice – a rare move for a cosmetic surgeon. Meanwhile Elliot, the urology specialist, undertook something equally out of the ordinary: mastering the cosmetic surgeon's liposuction procedure, so he too would be ready to extract and deploy ASC.

The procedure is simple enough that any physician with an MD degree, regardless of his or her chosen specialty, can easily perform it after undergoing a training session. Here's how it works: Patients undergo a mini-liposuction that yields the stromal vascular fraction (SVF), a protein-rich segment from processed adipose tissue. SVF contains a mononuclear cell line comprised mainly of autologous mesenchymal stem cells (fat derived and peri-vascular blood vessel derived stem cells), macrophage cells, endothelial cells, red blood cells, immune cells, and growth factors that facilitate the stem cell process and promote their activity. The fat sample is processed in a centrifuge in our treatment room as part of the surgical procedure; our technology enables us to isolate large numbers of viable cells, for optimal regenerative effect. The patient's SVF is then injected back into their body, either directly into the inflamed area (such as the knee or hip joint) or into the bloodstream, via an intravenous injection. When delivered by IV, the cells travel through the vascular system in search of areas of inflammation; the cells target those areas and then the damaged tissue activates the stem cells to begin the regeneration process.

Confident that we both had sufficient experience with this new method, Elliot came up with the idea to join our two practices – Mark's Beverly Hills office and Elliot's office in Rancho Mirage – and reincorporate both as branches of the California Stem Cell Treatment Center- dedicated to the investigational study of SVF. We set up our educational website www.Stemcellrevolution.com and in December of 2010, we treated our first patient at CSCTC. The first person to be treated with his own stem cells at the newly renamed facility was a Canadian businessman who'd endured neck and shoulder pain for many years; he had full resolution of his symptoms, and his success is durable to the present time. Like many of our patients, he later offered to invest in our clinic but we continue to remain privately owned in alignment with our philosophy to be physician owned and controlled. Because the service we offer is a totally closed procedure (the entire process is performed without exposure to the environment)– basically a therapeutic variation of Mark's perfected technique of extracting fat for cosmetic purposes – it is absolutely legal to perform since it is a type of lipo-transfer surgery. If it would be a laboratory procedure, it would not be FDA compliant, but it's not a laboratory procedure. We modified the technology to make it a surgical procedure instead of a laboratory procedure; we're one of only groups in the world doing it this way.

Other American facilities working with stem cells are laboratories, and all labs must be overseen by the FDA, to prevent disease transmission. This explains why the science pundits predict that stem cell practice won't be available for years to come. But because we perform closed surgical procedures on individual patients, we don't have to worry about communicable disease. What we're doing is not FDA-approved, yet it's FDA-compliant, completely legal, and available right now. We proudly follow the FDA's guidelines, but what we're doing is not under the FDA's jurisdiction because it's a closed surgical procedure. The FDA regulates drugs and medical devices but it is the respective State Medical Boards that regulate the "practice of medicine." As such, our protocol is no different than Mark extracting fat from his aesthetic patients and re-injecting it into their faces – and he's been doing that for almost 30 years. As we've proved with our own on-the-job training, any doctor is able to pick up the technique, no matter how general or specialized the practice s/he operates.

CSCTC is the first American medical practice to offer treatment with adipose derived stem cells in a methodical, investigative, academic, and organized manner. As the first to do this the way we do, initially we faced a great deal of criticism. We had to fly in the face of some peer issues, as competing clinics were located offshore and their quality was perceived as dodgy. Plus, we didn't have any funding, so we invested thousands of dollars of our own money and substantial time diverted from our own lucrative practices because we believed in what we were doing. Colleagues advised us to wait for peer-reviewed studies, otherwise we're "charlatans" and our treatment is so much "snake oil." But we saw no reason to delay putting this proven technology to work, to help people who need it and to educate as many other doctors as possible. We've been doing this for four years now, in a meaningful, controlled way, and we've treated more than 2,000 patients. If we evaluate a patient only to conclude that SVF wouldn't help the person, we won't treat that patient. We turn away as many as 20 percent of people who apply to us for treatment.

What CSCTC definitely does not do is culture cells to increase their strength in numbers. We cannot by law. Although cell culturing is currently par for the course in Spain, Russia, Sweden, Asia, and off-shore, here in the United States, if you grow (i.e. manipulate) cells, then by definition you become a drug manufacturer – and at that point you're under the auspices of the FDA. Culturing cells is beyond the scope of minimal manipulation, so growing is, for now, verboten. Hopefully, that restriction will soon change, as the ability to culture cells will permit American doctors to perform life-saving procedures such as generating custom, rejection-proof donor organs seeded with the transplant recipient's own cells (as Dr. Paolo Macchiarini did when he achieved the world's first tissue-engineered trachea transplant in Barcelona in 2008). Once an organization demonstrates FDA approved Good Manufacturing Practices (GMP) to culture (i.e. replicate and increase the numbers of cells), thus avoiding risk of disease transmission, then your own cells will eventually be available in even greater numbers. You will eventually bank your cells and get huge returns with interest. This brings possibilities are nearly unlimited such as creating your own individual lines of stem cells that could later be used not only for repair work but also to fight cancers since our stem cells have the ability to bring cancer therapies directly to damaged tissue where malignancies are growing. Many labs around the world are now looking at exploiting the cancer homing and identifying properties of stem cells and this area of stem cell science is attracting a lot of attention and interest today.

OK, we had "lightning in a bottle." We could have kept our technology proprietary by operating a niche clinic to help our patients exclusively, but our vision was to make regenerative therapies readily available to people who need them most, while rapidly increasing our ability to perform studies for safety and efficacy. Our hope was that someday, perhaps we could modify the way health care would be delivered in this country. In 2012, we made the decision to reach out to research partners and collaborate to spread the technology in a controlled fashion by starting the Cell Surgical Network to train research partners to collaborate on protocols and collect data together. If we selected key physicians who could participate in our investigative studies, and we conveyed our intellectual property freely to those physicians, then we could help even more people, and more rapidly advance the field.

Ultimately, it was our wish that patients could benefit from cell therapy without million-dollar labs, inaccessible university programs, expensive and inconvenient travel, regulatory hurdles, or bureaucratic obstacles. All we had to do was move stem cell rich tissues from areas of abundance to tissues that were damaged and therefore in need of additional stem cells to effect healing. Just physicians treating their patients with one more tool in the armamentarium to battle disease and accelerate healing, the way physicians have treated their patients for centuries. Wasn't this what we were taught when we took the Hippocratic oath? If we have a treatment that is apparently safe and effective, are we not at least ethically obligated to provide it for our patients? Are we not also obligated to teach it to our fellow physicians?

So, if it was that easy, not to mention legal, to establish an American stem cell clinic, then why hadn't it been done before? Most likely because specialists from different disciplines rarely collaborate and work together with a common therapeutic goal. We've had patients tell us that we're very "un-doctor-like" – and we take that as a compliment. And because we've never advertised – patients find us through word of mouth, physician referral, or by happening upon our Web site – another compliment we often hear is, "You guys are not commercial – I like that." Initially, Mark's patients were surprised when a cosmetic surgeon offered orthopedic treatment, while Elliot's patients were astonished to see a urologist performing liposuction.

Today, collaborating with our colleagues in different medical specialties, we offer treatment for conditions that are quite different from our original specialties, including heart disease, neurological disease, and muscular dystrophy. Patients with Hashimoto's Thyroiditis might be surprised to learn that there's a promising new treatment for this disease – however, they might not get the news from an endocrinologist, per se, but from a distinguished orthopedic surgeon with an interest in endocrinology! (He's Dr. Lawrence Schrader of the Cell Surgical Network, who expanded his practice to include stem cell therapy for a range of conditions far outside his original specialty; we'll meet him in the next chapter).

Today, the Cell Surgical Network we started in 2012 to teach other physicians has grown into an international organization that not only promotes cell therapy, but also treats actual patients using their own stem cells, harvested from their own fat. The team of highly qualified doctors we've formed is a bit out of the ordinary in that it's not based on a single specialty; we're a multi-specialty group, which you don't customarily see. Patients tell us they're amazed to discover doctors currently providing stem cell treatment – a service supposedly very complicated and still five or ten years off. While we faced arguments about the limitations of SVF, scientific studies and actual investigational patient treatments have demonstrated far more abilities for cell repair than we originally thought existed. Several of our patients have graciously agreed to share their stories to help illustrate these findings. SVF has provided us with a spectacular journey – bridging multiple disciplines, bringing many of us back to the joy of treating a variety of medical problems and often positively impacting our patients when little or no hope existed.

Chapter 2

AESTHETICS TO THERAPEUTICS

A plastic surgery practice might be the last place you'd expect to find relief from an orthopedic issue. But a plastic surgery practice – specifically, Mark's office in Beverly Hills – is exactly where many patients suffering from joint degeneration and arthritis experienced an end to months and even years of discomfort and diminished quality of life. Most of these patients had already taken multiple treatments – e.g. NSAID (non-steroidal anti-inflammatory) pain medications, steroid injections, hyaluronic acid injections, and even arthroplasty – yet they didn't get better. After intra-joint injection of SVF, on the other hand, most showed improvement, with many reporting "no more pain." Initially, we were as pleasantly surprised as our patients that a cosmetic surgery technique – liposuction – could yield such consistently effective therapeutic results. Today, the majority of our patients – and some of our most compelling success stories – are people with orthopedic problems who are happy to resume favorite activities many thought they'd have to give up permanently.

With any new medical technology, the first patients who step forward to try it out are trailblazers no less than the scientists who invent it. That's why we at CSCTC have enormous respect for the first two patients to undergo our treatment protocol in 2010. The very first was Laurie, who dealt with continual pain in her left knee as a result of a nasty ski accident followed by arthroscopic surgery to try and straighten out her damaged cartilage. At 37, she didn't want another failed arthroscopy – and she certainly didn't look forward to a total joint replacement at such a young age. Laurie loved hiking, but lately there wasn't enough Motrin to ease the pain. Her work also keeps Laurie on her feet most of the day; she is one of the anesthetists at Mark's plastic surgery practice in Beverly Hills, and she's terrific at her job. A strong lady with a stoic streak, she's never one to complain. In fact, if Mark hadn't mentioned his interest in investigating fat-derived stem cells, Laurie might never have mentioned the chronic pain she was suffering. She would've just kept it to herself.

However, if you were to have a look at Laurie's knee, it wouldn't take any medical experience to understand how badly damaged it had been. The joint felt like a sack of granola. You could practically hear the cartilage particles rubbing together and breaking apart. Laurie became patient number one in Mark's trial of adipose-derived stromal vascular fraction (SVF). But before Mark could perform the procedure on Laurie, it was necessary to have her evaluated by an orthopedic surgeon. Mark turned to Dr. Thomas Grogan of Santa Monica, one of the best, most solid orthopedic surgeons in the country. "If Grogan told me to go pound sand, and that he wouldn't consider an SVF injection, that would have possibly ended my pursuit of SVF administration for therapeutic conditions," Mark recalls. "I plied Tom with multiple articles that supported the use of adipose- and bone marrow-derived cells for the treatment of a variety of inflammatory and degenerative orthopedic conditions. All I asked is that he evaluate the patients that I referred to him, and then consider injecting the appropriate joint with cells that I took and prepared from my patients. Fortunately, he agreed."

After he assessed Laurie's knee, Dr. Grogan agreed that she had little to lose in trying an SVF injection. Of course, the first time is rarely the charm, as we still needed to work out kinks with the technique of harvesting and producing the SVF from fat. During that first procedure, Mark harvested fat from Laurie's abdomen without any difficulty. The early technique for producing SVF while discarding fat lacked the finesse and sophistication of our current techniques – call it version 1.0 – but we still managed to produce SVF. Dr. Grogan injected the SVF into Laurie's knee after performing a sterile prep and adding some local anesthesia to prevent pain. Still, Laurie reports, the injection "really hurt," as she felt a lot of pressure and pain on the injection. This was not a good sign, but the pain rapidly subsided and over the next few days her knee actually started feeling better, with less pain. Laurie started hiking again, and noticed that she could move about with greater ease.

While she seemed to respond very well to SVF, Laurie felt she had overdone it with the hiking, and didn't believe she gave herself enough opportunity to heal properly. This initial deployment was done in March 2010. By the end of that year, Mark had made several adjustments to the technique, which improved the procedure significantly. Roche Laboratories was now providing a medical-grade collagenase, and Mark revamped and modified the entire system in order to make it a completely closed, absolutely sterile, surgical procedure. Additionally, he added a filtration procedure that assured that we could not possibly add any debris or particles to the SVF that might be capable of forming clots within the patient's body or blood stream. So, in December 2010, we repeated the procedure on Laurie, with Dr. Grogan injecting her knee again. Between this and Laurie's first SVF experience, we had injected nearly 20 other patient's joints, and nearly all of them were relatively pain-free, but Laurie's injection still hurt her a lot. Laurie also had a strange condition she'd developed a few years earlier called RSD – reflex sympathetic dystrophy. This caused her to experience strange pains in her left arm and hand, especially when subjected to cold conditions. So, to address this, she also received intravenous SVF at the same time as her knee injection.

Several weeks later, Mark's cell phone rang; it was Laurie, excitedly exclaiming that she'd been skiing Montana without pain – bending and making turns just as she'd been able to do years ago, before her ski injury. As a bonus, the RSD seemed to have disappeared as well. Simply ecstatic, Laurie felt the second treatment was considerably improved, and she felt confident that she'd given her knee a better opportunity to heal without undue force before resuming serious exercise and ski activities. Nearly a year later, her medial (inside part of the knee) seemed to be completely healed, but the lateral (outside) area still had some crepitus (those creaking granola sounds), and some tenderness too. Mark provided Laurie an injection directly into the lateral compartment this time, and within weeks she felt fine. In fact, at her last exam, there was smooth motion and no crepitus at all. Laurie got her knee back and got rid of her RSD. By the time we'd done her last two treatments, we felt we really had the system down – but this didn't, and still doesn't, mean we could claim to cure everyone or anyone. As the chapters of this book will show, we've been investigating autologous (your own) SVF deployments for a variety of conditions, primarily to show that it is safe, and secondarily, to gather data to ascertain trends in effectiveness. Not every case we've seen had the favorable outcomes depicted in these chapters but we thought this cross section of our patient's stories is representative of the astonishing things we have seen since we started this project. Mark and I have been practicing surgeons for 60 years collectively and we both concur that our SVF project has been the most professionally rewarding time in our lives.

Mark wouldn't refer the next patient to Dr. Grogan until August 2010; the subject was an avid runner since her college days. She'd completed several marathons, and ran six miles every day. There are those among us that enjoy exercise, but this patient loved to run. Of course, even the most avid runners have only a limited amount of running left in their joints after a certain age, and this young lady of 56 had already logged enough miles for someone 100 years old. Three and half years prior to the time Mark referred her to Dr. Grogan on this occasion, she'd been experiencing left hip pain (we say "on this occasion" because she'd already been seeing Dr. G for trials of various anti-inflammatory medications, as well as a cortisone injection). Nothing seemed to be working, and now the thought of a total hip replacement, although not imminent, became a real consideration. Oh, by the way, this patient was Mark's wife, Saralee. So far, he didn't have to dig too deep into the patient pool to find prospective subjects for SVF trials.

Mark hadn't set up any formal protocols yet; he just wanted to see if SVF really worked. Could it live up to the success stories we'd heard from several scattered clinics around the world, including a few in the USA? If it did work, we had a unique and simple platform from which to prepare it. Saralee was the perfect patient to work with. She's what we call an informed patient, especially when it comes to orthopedics: She'd worked as a radiology technician and managed an orthopedics practice, so she could read X-rays with no problem. Now that she was the orthopedic patient, she could clearly see the degenerative changes in her own hip. Originally, Dr. Grogan had planned to inject

Saralee's hip after Mark produced the cells, but he had a scheduling conflict with another surgery, so he referred us to Dr. David Allegra at Resolution Imaging. After doing the mini-liposuction procedure under straight local anesthesia and preparing the cells – this time with a better technique, using a medical grade collagenase – Mark drove with Saralee a couple miles to the radiology office.

While Mark hoped Saralee would be seen and injected right away, there ended up being nearly an hour and a half delay. Meanwhile, Mark's got 6 cc's (just over a teaspoon) of Saralee's SVF solution sitting in a syringe in his shirt pocket; he couldn't decide whether to keep the solution cool or at a physiologic temperature – i.e. his! "I supposed I should've been worried at that point," Saralee recalls with a laugh. "I mean, it does sound pretty out-there. But I knew Mark would never do anything stupid. It's my job to play devil's advocate, as all husbands and wives do with each other. But Mark has always been so conservative that I completely trusted him." Dr. Allegra got Saralee set up on an X-ray table and took a quick shot of her hip. He then numbed her up with a local anesthetic, cleansed the area with a sterile prep, and draped the area off. He skillfully inserted a long needle into the area while checking its position with fluoroscopy (X-ray). He injected a little dye to confirm the proper location, and then Mark handed him the SVF, and Dr. Allegra injected that into the hip joint. And that was that. Saralee walked out of there. She resumed her normal activities the very next day, including light exercise on the stationary bike; the only workout routine she postponed was a return to running. Without remembering exactly when, but within a few weeks after receiving the injection, Saralee noticed that she'd wake up without the hobbling discomfort she'd resigned herself to feeling every morning upon getting out of bed. A month or so later, Saralee and Mark flew to Boston to visit their son, who was attending college there. As Mark recalls, "Saralee walked off the airplane and she turned to me and exclaimed, 'I have no pain – I don't feel anything in my hip. This is crazy!'" Crazy good: Mark gave Saralee a follow-up deployment of SVF a year after that, and today, four years later, she continues to remain pain-free. She avoided running because she didn't want to re-injure her hip; so she took up SoulCycle "because," she says, "I feel it's kinder and gentler to the body than running." She still works out for an hour each day without any discomfort. "My hip was excruciating," Saralee recalls. "Just lying in bed, it was killing me. I'm pain-free now. For two or three years, when traveling, my husband would get way ahead of me at airports because I'd be limping along – my hip was that stiff from sitting. Now, ever since that trip to Boston right after my first SVF injection, I'll walk off a plane after sitting for hours, no problem. And each time it hits me: *Wow, I'm back to normal.* That is huge! On a day-to-day basis, I completely forget that I ever even had pain."

Encouraged by reasonably successful outcomes with his anesthetist and his wife, Mark began telling patients about the wonders of their fat. "Indeed, it helped me better understand the aging process," Mark says, "and not only why fat grafting was useful and important to reverse the appearance of aging, but also how it actually worked." This exciting information came up time and again as Mark's cosmetic patients would inquire about liposuction or facial rejuvenation procedures. Joyce, 68, was anxious to find out how Mark proposed to help her stave off the ravages of facial aging. Several years previously, she had undergone a procedure for which Mark gained popularity or notoriety (depending on whom you talked to and when he had done the procedure). "What I call 3D stem cell/fat grafting these days has been widely known as fat grafting, fat transfer, lipo-transfer, fat injections, and the space lift," Mark explains. "Joyce had it done with good results several years prior, and as time marches on, eventually it needs to be repeated."

"I hoped it would be longer lasting or permanent," Joyce lamented.

"Unfortunately," Mark explained, "even the placement of permanent materials doesn't give a permanent result."

"How's that so?" she queried.

Mark had an "*Aha*" moment. "After all these years, I actually understood how we age, so I explained it to Joyce," he recalls. "Our fat cells live seven to ten years, then die off. They can be replaced by stem cells that turn into new fat cells, but eventually they run out and our face simply loses volume, so our skin appears to sag. So, even if you put in a permanent filler material, eventually you would lose fat cells and you'd end up with skin sagging over your filler material."

Joyce wanted to know: "If my facial fat is dissipating and running out of stem cells, why doesn't that happen elsewhere in my body?"

"It actually does," Mark explained. "If you are lucky enough not to die of heart disease, cancer, or getting hit by a bus, then eventually you simply run out of cells. Your abdomen, hips, and thighs are simply blessed with so many more fat cells and, consequently, stem cells, that it takes much longer to deplete these cells. Of course, if you live long enough, even these cells become depleted. We don't really find people over 100 with significant fat deposits. All of our organs are made up of cells, and all cells have a life expectancy. Our available reparative stem cells dwindle with age and simply can't keep up with the needs to replace our vital organ cells as they continue to fail. Eventually, we all run out of cells to the point we just don't have enough to sustain life."

"The good news," Mark added, "is that until we are very old – well past our eighties – most of our body fat remains loaded with stem cells and now, we can actually isolate these cells from fat – and not only use them to help improve facial contours, but also for therapeutic applications, such as repairing arthritis and other orthopedic conditions."

Suddenly, Joyce leaned forward and exclaimed, "Wait, can you fix my knees? I'm scheduled to have a total knee replacement next month and I'd do anything to avoid surgery."

Mark went on to explain how he'd been working with Dr. Tom Grogan, a leading orthopedic surgeon, on a very preliminary investigative project. If Dr. Grogan found her to be a reasonable candidate, Mark could perform a mini-liposuction procedure under straight local anesthesia and then prepare her cells by separating them from her fat. These cells – what we call SVF or stromal vascular fraction – could then be injected into the joint to help it regenerate damaged tissue. The one-day procedure would be completed within two hours. Instead of scheduling a fairly lucrative facial cosmetic procedure, Joyce made an appointment with Dr. Grogan, and soon we performed an investigative trial of SVF injections on her knees at mere cost. As she was one of the early patients in this trial, we just wanted to cover our expenses until we had evidence that this really worked. Well, once again, it did work, just as it had with Laurie and Saralee. Joyce's pain cleared up fairly quickly, and she became progressively more comfortable moving about. But would it last?

Two years later, Joyce had an appointment with Mark. He walked into the exam room expecting to hear that her knees hurt, her face had aged, or there was some new problem. Instead, she told him that she just wanted to thank him, because her knees continued to be pain-free after all this time. She felt better and simply needed to express her happiness and gratitude for helping her avoid a more invasive and significant operation. So, how did a cosmetic surgeon shift his focus from necks to knees? How did he get involved with SVF rich in stem cells, and start doing therapeutic treatments? And, how did he team with a urologist – Dr. Elliot Lander – to eventually form a company (California Stem Cell Treatment Center) and a network of doctors – the Cell Surgical Network – interested in applying this technology to help their patients? Shouldn't this be coming out of a university lab or big pharma? And are we really ready for clinical applications? Many of our critics think the answer to those last questions is, undoubtedly yes. They take issue, first and foremost, with the fact that CSCTC got its start in a plastic surgeon's office. Many people, both within and outside of the medical field, like to put down the specialty. And yet, without plastic surgery and its practitioners, we might never have discovered that adipose tissue – fat – holds such rich reserves of mesenchymal stem cells.

Back in the early 1980s, a group of cosmetic and plastic surgeons toured Europe as a contingency to learn about a new and growingly popular procedure called lipolysis. An Italian doctor, Giorgio Fischer, and his father, developed a technique for removing fat through a type of suction and cleaving procedure. Eventually, it caught on in France, where Yves-Gerard Illouz used a strong suction machine alone to remove unwanted fat. Another Frenchman, Pierre Fournier, discovered that you could remove the unwanted fat with a simple syringe harvesting technique. Among the contingency of doctors to have visited was a young man named Michael Elam, who almost jokingly referred to the technique as liposuction. In doing so, he originated the term that Julius Newman would widely popularize.

As a young surgeon, having completed a residency in otolaryngology/ head and neck surgery (also commonly referred to as ENT or ear, nose and throat), Mark attended one of the first major U.S. courses on liposuction. This group that toured Europe organized the meeting that they presented in Century City, California, in January 1984. At that time, Mark saw himself as a facial plastic surgeon and intended to apply liposuction to areas around the face, particularly for those with an overly fatty submental (below the chin) area. During this same meeting, two groups of cosmetic physicians agreed to amalgamate their societies and as such, they formed the American Academy of Cosmetic Surgery. In those days, cosmetic procedures were still largely considered something to be learned outside of a traditional residency program. Of course, that made sense as these elective procedures were not covered by insurance policies, and thus didn't easily fit into teaching programs that were essentially subsidized by government and, occasionally, private insurance financing. During Mark's residency, he and his colleagues had the good fortune to set up their own resident clinic for cosmetic facial procedures and amassed very significant numbers of cosmetic cases, often with the tutelage of some of the finest ENT and plastic cosmetic surgeons in the Los Angeles area. For just $1,000, a patient could get a face lift and more from senior residents supervised by the likes of Kurt Wagner or Morey Parkes, two of the giants of the Beverly Hills cosmetic surgery scene.

As there were a limited number of doctors performing body liposuction in those days, Mark's patients asked if he could also do body liposuction. Having been trained in general surgery prior to his head and neck residency, it wasn't difficult for Mark to incorporate these "soft tissue" procedures into his practice, even though they were below the clavicle. Of course, head and neck surgeons deal with soft tissues, even ones below the clavicle – they just mainly fix things above the clavicle even if they harvest tissues from down under. Within a short time, Mark became fairly adept at liposuction and offered it along with his other procedures.

Not long after the advent of liposuction, Mark attended a meeting in Philadelphia in 1986 where Pierre Fournier, one of the fathers of liposuction, declared that he had taken some of his own liposuctioned fat and had successfully injected it into his own forehead. "Voila," he declared, "I have a lump." More lights turned on, and before you knew it, plastic surgeons were performing or trying to perform fat grafting by injecting fat harvested by liposuction. Even with a host of studies, early attempts were marginal at best and to this day, while it always works, there is a degree of variability from patient to patient. Eventually, during the early 90's, Mark realized that while there may have been a lot of skepticism about fat grafting, there was no doubt that he and his colleagues had mis-diagnosed the main causes of aging and attributed it mostly to gravitational changes on the skin. Thus, all cosmetic procedures had been aimed at lifting. Mark and a number of his colleagues began looking at aging in a three-dimensional way. Ultimately, they came to understand that the appearance of facial aging was largely due to the loss of facial fat. "It would be my later work in the arena of fat derived stem cells that would eventually clarify the true nature of aging – namely, that we are made up of dozens of trillions of cells, and that these cells eventually die," Mark says. "Fat cells, for example, generally live 7 to 10 years before they die off."

In April 2008, Dr. Hee Young Lee and his team from Seoul, South Korea brought his "Lipokit" machine to Mark's office to demonstrate how they prepared fat for grafting. The whole preparation process could be performed in a very neat and clean manner. Indeed, the entire process remained a completely closed, sterile, surgical procedure. The fat was optimally harvested and prepared while eliminating dead or broken cells, local anesthesia, blood and any unnecessary debris. Mark bought the machine that day – one of the first two machines even sold in the U.S. – and soon emerged as a leading practitioner of the fat-grafting technique, with patients seeking him out to rejuvenate their faces and augment their breasts. In the name of surgically enhancing beauty, fat had come to be viewed, not as something to get rid of, but rather, as something valuable to harvest, to combat the aging process. Ultimately, fat would be viewed for what it was all along: a rich source of mesenchymal stem cells.

On a trip to Japan, Mark attended a lecture on stem cells given by Dr. Kotaro Yoshimura, a plastic surgeon and one of the leading researchers working with fat-derived stem cells. Regardless of his or her specialty, a doctor couldn't sign up for a better post-graduate course anywhere in the world, and Mark was blown away. Dr. Yoshimura helped his colleagues to understand how significant these cells were, how they worked, and how doctors could work with them. As a plastic surgeon, Dr. Yoshimura kept his focus on the cells' plastic surgical applications. But the more Mark thought of fat-derived stem cells and their therapeutic potential, the more he wanted to spread the wealth beyond the strictly aesthetic concerns of his chosen surgical discipline. Fat was the missing link: the most natural material with which to correct problems caused by aging in the body, not just the face. The three-dimensional approach to plastic surgery that Mark had espoused now gave him a different approach to the practice of medicine. Just as he'd tried to improve the treatment of the aging face, he wondered why other aging parts – notably, the joints – couldn't also benefit from stem-cell-rich fat.

Meanwhile, Elliot was determined to apply the healing potential of fat-derived stem cells for his patients, many of whom struggled with conditions for which there is no cure, only management of pain. Shortly after Mark and Dr. Grogan teamed up to treat orthopedic patients with their own stem cells, we – Elliot and Mark – partnered to incorporate the multispecialty California Stem Cell Treatment Center, with the goal of further investigating the tremendous potential of SVF for various health issues in addition to orthopedics.

Over the last few years, we've continued training doctors, mostly surgical specialists or teams with multiple specialists. It's one thing to turn out improved results within your own practice, but our colleagues rewarded us by effectively recapitulating our findings in their own practices.

As an example, our colleague Dr. Lawrence Schrader, founder of Schrader Orthopedics in Cordova, Tennessee, became an officially trained affiliate of the California Stem Cell Treatment Center in 2012. During his two-day training session, Larry also underwent SVF treatment with us. Larry's achievements as an orthopedic surgeon are well known in his field, where he's sought-after for his knee pain expertise, but equally impressive are his athletic achievements, and his recovery from an early sports injury.

Larry had been an accomplished athlete and track-and-field star since high school, with a history of heavy weight lifting. As a teenager, he sustained a torn meniscus. The menisci are the two C-shaped cartilages that protect the knee joint from stress, whether it's due to everyday walking or aerobic athletic activity. A meniscus can tear from trauma caused by twisting or hyper-flexing the knee joint. Larry underwent old-fashioned orthopedic surgery to repair the meniscus while still in school (this was back before arthroscopy was a thing). Then, in college, he was on the track team and became a discus thrower; when one particularly motivating coach mentioned that a hammer thrower was needed, Larry volunteered. At 5'11 he was on the short side for the hammer throw – which happens to be one of the oldest competitions in the Olympic Games – but he was determined to master this new athletic challenge. In no time, Larry got so good at the sport that he was competing in national championships by the end of his freshman year. "There's a lot of leg work involved," he explains, "plus the hammer itself weighs sixteen pounds, and you exert a lot of force in throwing. Being small, I did a lot of weight lifting with my legs," he adds. "I would do squats up to 700 pounds, to try to make up for my lack of height."

All that action took a toll on Larry's right knee, which was already compromised by the meniscal tear. Like many collegiate athletes who enter the medical field, Larry decided to practice orthopedic medicine. The hammer figured in that discipline too, he explains: "Orthopedic surgery is very straightforward mechanical engineering. You basically hammered in, or hammered out, something that had gotten stuck. We used to have a saying: If it doesn't fit, get a bigger hammer – and if it still doesn't fit, get a bigger surgeon!" Meanwhile, his own knee provided a fine example of how, once a joint is subjected to continuous wear and tear, it grows progressively weaker. "All through my medical residency," Larry recalls, "I had a whole, nice series of X-rays of my knee getting worse over the years." That didn't stop him from continuing to compete in track and field until age 50, representing at several world championships. In fact, awareness of his vulnerable point fine-tuned his orthopedic practice; Larry became renowned as a knee specialist. By now, however, his own knee was getting "more and more arthritic," he says. "I have a family, and one of our main activities together was snow skiing – but it got to the point where I couldn't put pressure on my knees. So I decided to try and snowboard at 50. Well, if you start learning to snowboard at 50, you fall a lot – and that's how I ended up tearing up my shoulders. As you compensate for one torn shoulder, you tear up the other one. With both shoulders painful and weak, I had trouble sleeping."

Meanwhile, the right knee that had bothered him since high school became so unstable, Larry recalls, "I had trouble sitting down in a chair." Finally, in 2012, he scheduled for himself the same procedure he'd performed hundreds of times for patients, as frequently as five times per week: a partial knee replacement. Three weeks prior to his knee surgery, Larry traveled to our Rancho Mirage office for a training session with several other surgeons. During the demonstration, we ask our colleagues if they'd like to volunteer to undergo the SVF harvesting and injection. Just as he had when his college coach needed a hammer thrower, Larry stepped up without hesitation. "I went there with two bad shoulders and a bad knee," he says. "I was really intrigued that so many conditions, systemic or in the joints, could be helped by something minimally invasive. It's such an easy harvesting technique, and almost risk-free – the only thing you need to worry about is sterility." After procuring SVF containing stem cells, we make a practice of routinely counting all of our samples for quality assurance, to check for viability and appearance before deploying (injecting) it into patients. Testing showed that Larry's fat yielded an abundance of cells in his SVF, so after we finished injecting his shoulders, we asked if there was anything else he might want treated. He mentioned his impending surgery, but said he wanted us to inject the knee anyway. So that's what we did. "I didn't think anything about it," Larry remembers. "I've injected my own knee a million times." About an hour later, our visiting colleagues joined us for dinner. "How does your knee feel?" one of his fellow doctors asked Larry, who replied, "Why do you ask?"

Larry experienced the same phenomenon Saralee had described: When chronic joint pain finally goes away, it doesn't take long to become a distant memory. "For the first time in years, I hadn't thought about it because it didn't hurt," Larry recalls. "I started moving the knee around, got up and did some deep knee bends. It surprised me that the pain was gone. But that response has been close to universal in the patients I've treated for knee pain with their own stem cells." That night, his now pain-free shoulders allowed Larry to enjoyed a restful night's sleep.

Three weeks after returning home, he went ahead with his scheduled partial knee replacement surgery; he went skiing with his family two months later, "with really no limitation," he reports. The shelf life of a partial knee replacement is twenty years, and as Larry points out, "two years of response is nothing compared to a twenty-year follow-up." Still, looking back on it, would he have done anything differently? "I would've given it more time, no question," he says. "Being symptom-free for three weeks at that point in time, I would have put the surgery on hold if I hadn't already scheduled it. It's like I always tell my patients: If I can relieve your pain, you don't need surgery. I've treated eight patients with stem cells for their knees, and the pain went away for all but one. When the other seven patients stood up, they reported their pain was gone. That's pretty amazing. And when I've taken follow-up X-rays, four to six to eight months to a year later, I've seen cartilage thickness growing back in the knees."

In short order, Larry renamed his Tennessee practice the Schrader Orthopedics and Stem Cell Treatment Center; among his satisfied patients are his wife and two of their three children. "Everybody asks for treatment and results – and pretty much everybody responds," Larry concludes. "Another thing I commonly find in treating patients is they've got a few other things going on that suddenly get better: problems with Crohn's or digestive issues, or ten years of back pain. I've treated people with brain and balance problems, where they couldn't speak well, and after an SVF injection, their speech and balance literally improved. So I tell my prospective stem cell patients there are lots of side effects – and almost all of them are good."

Chapter 3

HEART OF THE MATTER

Cardiac disease, as the leading cause of death in the United States, claims the lives of 600,000 people every year and thus represents one of the most important areas of investigational stem cell therapy. As scientists and physicians, we're not supposed to get too excited about anything, but it would be tough not to get excited about the applications of stem cell therapy to heart disease. The heart – that muscular organ essential to the body's survival – responds very well to treatment with adult stem cells. Stem cells are proving to be very effective in treating cardiomyopathy (congestive heart failure), a chronic weakening of heart muscle function, that historically meant a death sentence for those unlucky enough to receive the diagnosis.

Made up of muscle tissue, the heart works like a pump, stimulated by electrical currents to pump blood through the blood vessels to all parts of the body. In cardiomyopathy patients, the heart muscle weakens and cannot function normally. As the heart loses function, it also enlarges in size. As a result, the heart is increasingly unable to do its job, causing other body parts to lose function too. Ultimately, the patient dies of heart failure – but first, he or she experiences a kind of slow, protracted death, with some or all of the terrifying symptoms of heart failure, including shortness of breath, fatigue, swelling of the ankles, feet, and legs (due to edema, which is buildup of fluid in the tissues), dizziness, light-headedness, fainting, chest pain, heart murmurs, and arrhythmias (irregular heartbeats). With cardiomyopathy, quality of life is comparable to metastatic cancer: You can't breathe properly; you have no energy. It's a miserable way to exist. As the final insult, cardiomyopathy also carries an eighty percent mortality rate. And yet, early studies seem to indicate that, after a simple IV infusion of mesenchymal cells, the heart muscle begins to contract and do its job better, growing stronger with each beat.

We reckoned that SVF would have a similar effect in getting damaged hearts to pump with greater efficiency – and we got compelling validation of our theory after treating several cardiac patients, who have all emerged from treatment to beat the cardiomyopathy odds. One of those patients is Kalani Skinner. For Kalani, yard work is not a chore to be avoided or procrastinated – it's a measure of wellness, and a heart-healthy workout he looks forward to doing three times a week. "It's part of my cardiac rehab," explains the former doctor of chiropractic, who has also worked many years at a hospital as a registered nurse. "I don't go to a traditional gym anymore," he adds. "I do yard work." Except he's not talking about raking leaves: "It's heavy manual labor: I use a chain saw to cut down trees and brush, a tree limb saw and a pole saw, a weed whacker to cut down grass, picks and shovels to dig up roots or clean out shrubs that are too big for hand-held shears." The trees he's describing are not small saplings – many of them are imposing redwoods. Where Kalani lives – in the mountains outside San Francisco, ten miles from the Big Basin National Park, where forest fires are a sadly common occurrence – yard work is literally do or die: "The Fire Department requires us all to maintain a fire break and to keep our gutters clean," Kalani says. "So I work pretty hard." Just a few years ago, however, yard upkeep presented an almost insurmountable physical challenge. "I would wake up feeling like a truck ran over me," he recalls. "I couldn't carry a bag of fertilizer uphill. So I didn't even attempt it, because I knew it would be too heavy of a work load."

That's because a few years ago, Kalani's heart was giving out. In January of 2000, he was treating patients at his busy chiropractic practice, where his specialty was sports medicine. In addition to helping his athletic patients improve their running game to perform their best, Kalani was quite active himself, logging between 18 and 22 miles of running each week. But one morning, he recalls, "I thought I had the flu. I had a cough, and my symptoms had been going on for two days. My receptionist said, 'This is more than the flu' – my legs were swollen."

After a chest X-ray at his doctor's office, Kalani, then 46, was admitted to the hospital intensive care unit. His receptionist's hunch had been correct: Kalani did not have the flu; he was, in fact, in the midst of a life-changing cardiac event. The diagnosis: idiopathic cardiomyopathy, or weakened heart muscle causing congestive heart failure. "My heart was as large as a football," Kalani says. "My cardiac output [ejection fraction] was 10 percent; normal is 60. I was in heart failure." The renowned cardiologist Dr. Jackie See, our colleague and founding member of our treatment team, explains the EF this way: "We cardiologists are number freaks, and we have this number called the ejection fraction, which is the ratio of the heart when it's full of blood, to the heart after it's contracted. The lower the ejection fraction, the worse the prognosis, and the earlier the death. This was described at Harvard when I was a research fellow there in the 1970s, so we've known it for a long time, but we didn't know what to do about it."

Having worked full-time as a registered nurse in the intensive care cardiac surveillance unit at a nearby hospital, looking after people with tachycardia and lethal arrhythmias, Kalani was familiar with cardiology in general and cardiomyopathy in particular – but never expected his own heart would give out on him. Fitted with a pacemaker-defibrillator, he says, "I found myself in the role of patient, just like the people I'd cared for." For the next eight years, from 2000 to 2008, "I was slowly maintaining a cardiac output of 30-38," Kalani says. "I was doing my due diligence as a cardiac patient, staying on a regular exercise program, riding my bicycle because I couldn't run or get my heart rate up too high without risking going into cardiac dysrhythmia [irregular heartbeat]. Bicycling was a difficult effort, but it was not as traumatic as running. I was also able to do yoga. I got plenty of exercise and sleep, stopped drinking alcohol, and made some dietary changes; I ate and juiced vegetables, and quit eating bacon." In 2004, Kalani was obliged to close his chiropractic practice due to economic factors. "It was impossible to compete with the Silicon Valley for office space, which starts at $7.50 a square foot," he says. So he went to work full-time as a cardiac cath lab nurse, admitting patients coming into the hospital for angiograms, angioplasties, pacemaker implants, and electrophysiology, as well as teaching cardiac rehab. "I'm still doing that job," Kalani says, "although I keep my chiropractic license current. And there's no doubt that teaching cardiac rehab enhanced my survivability. People with a cardiac output of 10 or less statistically die of some catastrophic event within 30 months."

In 2008, Kalani developed coronary artery disease, and his first stent was installed. In 2010, his LAD (left anterior descending coronary artery) was found to be blocked by plaque. In 2013, after an episode of shortness of breath, he had another stent installed. In the meantime, Kalani became a patient of our esteemed colleague and founding member of our treatment team, the renowned cardiologist Dr. Jackie See. "My relationship with Dr. See also enhanced my survivability," Kalani says. "He's a very knowledgeable, loving soul, and his recommendations and alternative therapies helped me recover from my congestive heart failure event. He would examine me every three months, and work with my cardiologist. The fact that I maintained an ejection fraction of 38-40 is amazing, because if you look at the literature, statistically a person with my diagnosis will die within three years. Dr. See had me on branched chain amino acids and other nutritional interventions, including turmeric; he restricted my diet to eliminate sweets and keep my blood sugar low." Between his own interest in emerging alternative therapies and Dr. See's scholarship of regenerative medicine, it was inevitable that Kalani would seek out treatment with SVF. We treated him in July 2013. So, how's he doing now?

For starters, his ejection fraction went from 38 to a documented 60 percent! But let him tell you the details: "My heart has shrunk down; it's almost returned to its original size," Kalani says. "Although I still have heart enlargement, because as we age, the pump has to work harder to meet the body's demands, so it enlarges – it's a natural progression. There's scar tissue in my right ventricle, from the original heart failure and cardiomyopathy. My heart has benefited substantially from the autologous stem cell treatment. Before, I wasn't able to walk up a steep hill without feeling like a truck had run over me; now, I walk the hills around my house and I'm able to do physical work. I can carry a bag of fertilizer up a steep hill, and that was certainly something I couldn't do prior to my stem cell treatment. For a guy with all my health problems, I'm doing remarkably well – without the cells I got, I don't believe I would be doing as well as I am today. I felt different within two days of treatment. I can say that the stem cells helped me feel like I was all

27

rested on six hours of sleep, and that my general sense of well-being improved right away, and so did my work tolerance. I'll be out in the yard today for at least six hours. I'll be able to do that, then get a good night's sleep, then wake up and feel like I can get up and go do it again."

John Gregori is another one of our patients who is grateful for increased stamina, both in and out of the yard. John is not as famous as another very well-known cardiac patient, Dick Cheney; in fact, he's not famous at all. Yet he and the former Vice President have one critical thing in common: Cardiac disease qualified them both for heart transplantation. For more than ten years, John lived with non-ischemic dilated (congestive) cardiomyopathy, also known as heart muscle disease. John was experiencing all of the symptoms of cardiomyopathy, but wasn't diagnosed correctly until 2008. To look at him, you would never have guessed the gravity of his illness – it even escaped his doctors, at first. A bodybuilder all his life, John at age 49 had no problem bench-pressing 250 pounds, twenty times daily, an exercise routine that could easily defeat many men half his age, but one that never left John feeling tired. His lean, muscular physique – he's six foot two and 185 pounds – was more cowboy than cardiac patient. John's kids used to joke that he had "comic-book arms." Although happily married to the children's mother, his wife of 34 years, John was proud of being routinely "hit on by women in their 20s."

And yet, despite the workouts and killer abs, John was far from the picture of health. "I used to smoke cigarettes, a pack a day," he admits. "I started getting pains in my lungs and having trouble breathing. When I stopped smoking, the pain would go away, but when I started lighting up again, it would come back. My general practitioner told me I had emphysema, but kept wondering why inhalers weren't working for me." At the same time, John explains, "My bowels were so bad that I would spend four hours on the toilet every day. I was also peeing all night, so the doctor prescribed prostate medicine. We didn't know that it was really my heart all along. I had trouble breathing because my abdomen would fill up with water, crushing my lungs; my bowels and prostate were failing because not enough blood was getting down there."

The accurate diagnosis finally came when John needed an operation … on his hand. John's scheduled procedure – removal of bone spurs from an old injury sustained during his years working as a bulldozer mechanic – had to be performed under anesthesia, so his doctors ordered a routine echocardiogram (EKG) to determine whether or not it was safe to put him under. During an EKG, sound waves are used to show images of the heart and the blood pumping through it. The anesthesiologist saw nothing in John's EKG to raise concern, so John underwent the hand operation. "Within two weeks, I could hardly walk," John recalls. "I was limping because of a blood clot in my left leg. Then, a blood clot in my right hand turned my ring finger and middle finger black." A few days later, after undergoing more tests, John received very bad news. "The doctor called to tell me that I had some major blockage going on: a left bundle branch block," John says. "That means your heart is not receiving the signals telling it to beat." John had to get to the emergency hospital without delay. "They did an ultrasound and treadmill test. When I talked to the doctor, he said, 'You're a very sick man.'" John's ejection fraction was dangerously low: ten percent (a normal heart is 60 percent). "So at ten percent," John says with characteristic bluntness, "you're damn near dead. The doctor said he would put in a stent to open the blockage, and then I'd be 'as good as new.'" This procedure is called an angioplasty. "So I went in for the angio," John recalls, "and when I woke up, the doctor and nurse were standing over me. 'You need a heart transplant,' the doctor said." John's prognosis was grim: he didn't have more than a few years to live, at best. John, whose father had died of the disease at age 63, took the news hard, lying in bed "for days and days," he recalls.

"I was sick and I felt like shit," John recalls. "I couldn't do anything. I had to chop firewood for winter, which is pretty hard to do when you're dying of heart failure. I had maybe one good day a week, and six bad ones. Sometimes, I had two good and five bad days." However, upon receiving a correct diagnosis, he was able to stop taking prostate medication and using inhalers, with his doctor's OK. To prolong his heart's function, John was rigged with an implantable cardioverter defibrillator (ICD). A combination pacemaker-defibrillator, this electronic device is recommended for patients with severe cardiac failure. Inserted under the skin in the upper chest, near the collarbone, the ICD consists of a pulse generator containing a battery and a small computer, connected to specific parts of the heart with one or more lead wires. This device continuously monitors the heart's electrical activity, stimulating it to beat faster or slower until normal rhythm is restored. John also received low-tech cardiac benefits from the heart-healthy presence of his family's three Yorkshire terriers, who provided generous doses of comfort on days when he could barely function – days, he recalls, when "I couldn't walk twenty feet without sleeping six hours."

John soon became motivated to research his condition, and possible alternative treatments for it, online – on days when he had the energy for it, that is. Even with his name on the waiting list for a heart, John felt hopeless. Statistics show that some 300 people die each year waiting for a donor organ. What's more, John adds, "From my research online, I knew that when you get an organ transplant, your clock starts ticking even faster than with a failing heart – it leaves you open to all kinds of disease." John understood, correctly, a sad reality of organ transplantation: that transplant patients often succumb to cancer, because the immunosuppressive medication taken to prevent rejection of the donor organ weakens the body's own cancer-fighting ability. While he awaited a cure that, to him, seemed like just a different kind of death sentence, John stepped up his online research. "I decided to take my life into my own hands," he says. He remembers "stumbling onto stem cells" after seeing a television news feature on the subject.

Shortly after that, in 2011, John came across our Web site, StemCellRevolution.com, and wrote us a letter describing his situation and medical history. In no uncertain terms, he let us know how strong he is, and how fast he heals. After reviewing the application, we reached out to John and scheduled his procedure, which we performed on September 6, 2011. "For the first time, I had hope," John remembers. "Everywhere else I'd asked about stem cells – at universities that were conducting stem cell trials – I was told, 'We're sorry but we're not doing that right now.' It was so frustrating. It was like, 'If you need them, too bad!' Well, I wasn't letting somebody else decide my fate. I'll decide my own fate."

On the day of John's treatment, we also checked his testosterone. During his workup, we noted that his testosterone was low, and testosterone is proven to improve muscle function. The heart is a muscle, so we always advise our cardiomyopathy patients to optimize their testosterone levels. John's first treatment was directly into the heart, under general anesthesia. We don't do this anymore, because we've found that IV treatments, performed under local anesthesia, give excellent cardiac results. John's subsequent treatment in November 2012, and all our other cardiac treatments, have been IV only to this day. This makes treatment with stem cells far less invasive than most other cardiac procedures. About ninety days after treatment, John reports, "I started feeling good again. I felt like I was in my thirties – I could go weeks without feeling sick. My wife and I would make love for two hours every day!" Gradually, John had resumed his bodybuilding routine. He was also eagerly reaching for his axe, and splitting a quarter cord of firewood every day. "Before, I'd split a piece of wood and sit down to recover, then get up to split another," he says. "Now, here I was splitting one after another. It took me only an hour or two to do a quarter cord – enough to last about a week."

Calling himself "a firm believer in stem cells," John is astonished at the improvement cell therapy brought to his quality of life. "Before, I'd put on my shoes and walk from the bedroom to the front door – then have to go to bed for hours to recharge," he says. "Now I could go all day – and go really hard – before I needed a nap, so it was pretty amazing. Bodybuilding helped me too; whenever I started feeling crappy, I would work out and feel better." His daily workout routine today consists of four sets of 25 pushups. "I still do things around house – work in the yard, pick up plants, landscape, seed. As a retired mechanic, I can still change tires and work on my car – I just don't want to." John sings backup vocals with a Southern hard-rock band; "They're all professionals, I'm the weak link," he says with a laugh. But where his health is concerned, he's the headliner and the talent manager. Even when he doesn't expect to stay out late, he lets himself get plenty of rest. "I live a fairly normal life now," John says, "except for when I'm done for the day, *I am done* – even if that means taking a nap in the early evening, if I feel like I need to. Once in a while, I'll take an hour-long nap around 2 pm."

But John's biggest milestone was losing his place on the heart transplant waiting list. How did that happen? Because his ejection fraction went from ten percent to higher than 30 – so he no longer qualified for an urgent organ donation! Today, John experiences, he says, five great days and two bad ones per week – a big difference from the two "OK" days and five "terrible" ones that defined his average week prior to stem cell therapy. He experienced an unfortunate setback when, during a routine device check, a technician mistakenly switched on the rate response feature of his ICD, and his ejection fraction dropped to twenty percent. Although it caused John a great deal of discomfort – "It felt like some had just caught a trout, and it was flopping around inside my chest" – he was still no longer sick enough for the heart-transplant waiting list.

He may joke about having "bad hands and a bad heart," but we're confident that John's heart is in very good hands. "I don't eat crap anymore," he says. "When I was first diagnosed, it was like, zero salt, and I stuck with it religiously. Now, I'll let myself have pizza once in a while. I still eat a lot of fruit, and I take all kinds of supplements: potassium, L-arginine, L-carnitine, fish oil. I was taking CoQ10 when I was really sick, but I don't need it anymore." Perhaps most important, the cardiac patient who defied the odds makes a point of getting generous doses of heart-healthy TLC. He and his wife are more happily married than ever. "Let me put it to you this way: I was dying, so now, when I make love to my wife, it's like every day is her birthday and my last day on Earth – that's how I do it," he concludes. "It's very passionate, and I cherish every minute."

Chapter 4

JUST BREATHE

In an ideal world, breathing would come naturally to everyone – as naturally as pausing to listen to the beautiful Pearl Jam song "Just Breathe." But for the more than 18 million adults and 6.8 million children who struggle with asthma in America, every single breath is a result of serious effort – and that effort is exhausting over time. "Imagine having to do a lot of inhales just to take one breath," says Eddie Ortiz, who doesn't have to imagine what it's like to cope with asthma; he's been struggling with the disease since age 10. "I had it pretty bad for years – I could barely breathe," he recalls. "My Mom and Dad took me to the hospital when I had asthma attacks, and one time they almost lost me."

Children, especially, experience a diminished quality of life as a result of coping with asthma, a sad fact with which Eddie is also very familiar. "I used to play basketball, but I would get winded real quick, so as a player I was worthless – the other kids made fun of me all the time," he says. "They used to call me Wheezer – 'Here comes Wheezer,' they'd say, because I was always walking around wheezing. That really made me strong in a lot of ways," he adds. "Having a hard time breathing is something you learn how to deal with. You don't complain about it – you just deal with it."

Eddie "just dealt with it," uncomplaining, for more than 40 years. He'd tried medications and injections, with no success. "They didn't help at all, not one bit," he says, "and I hate inhalers." But after we successfully treated Eddie's wife Nancy for a knee injury she sustained in a car accident, Eddie became something of a cheerleader for adult stem cells. Seeing the change Nancy's treatment brought about in her quality of life motivated Eddie to tell many of their friends and neighbors about our practice, and we're grateful to him for the many referrals he sent our way.

But what about Eddie? He'd become so accustomed to a lifetime of shallow breathing that it took him some time to consider undergoing treatment himself. "I saw on the CSCTC Web site that the doctors treat asthma," Eddie says. "All the years I'd had asthma, I'd never heard of anybody saying they could treat it.". Put another way, there's a very good chance that asthma sufferers won't have trouble breathing after treatment with their own stem cells. Eddie's response to that was, "You're kidding me!" Despite his wife Nancy's success with the treatment, despite the many patients he sent to us, Eddie didn't become one of our patients himself for more than a year – that's how accustomed he was to "dealing with" asthma, and how skeptical he was that any treatment, even the stem cells he champions so vocally, could alleviate (remedy) a lifetime of shallow breathing.

The motivation to be treated came after Eddie – who is an avid internet researcher – learned that chronic asthma ultimately leads to congestive heart failure. Over time, the lungs cannot take in enough oxygen to keep the heart pumping properly. That information, together with the hope that he might experience what it's like to take a deep breath with ease, finally made Eddie decide to give stem cell therapy a try. We treated him in June 2013. Immediately following the procedure, Eddie recalls, "I didn't notice any difference in my breathing. Then Nancy and I left the Center and went to go get lunch around the corner. Maybe half an hour had gone by, when all of a sudden, I took a deep breath – it was the first time I ever took a deep breath."

Nancy recalls the moment: "We were eating salads at Sherman's Deli in Palm Springs. I said, 'Honey, how's your breathing?' And he took a deep breath and said, 'Oh my God, I can breathe!' Later, back at home, Eddie was delighted to awake at three in the morning. "I took a deep breath – a real deep breath," he says. "Normally, whenever I'd do that, I would cough immediately afterward. This time, I didn't have to cough. I woke Nancy up to tell her, 'I can breathe! It's an absolute miracle!' She said, 'Go to sleep!'" Since Eddie's procedure, both he and his wife have enjoyed more restful sleep. "He'd always had shallow breath, and even when we'd go to bed at night, he would snore and whistle," Nancy says. "I don't hear that whistling anymore."

The increased stamina Eddie has experienced since treatment enables him to stay in better shape physically. "I can walk a lot better now than I ever did before," he says. "I can walk for hours without getting tired or having any shortness of breath. Nancy and I walk a lot – it's the best exercise, but before, she couldn't walk for a while because of her knees, and I couldn't walk because of my asthma." Eddie is convinced that adult stem cell therapy did more than improve his breathing and his level of physical fitness: it actually saved his life.

Now, Eddie is even more vocal than ever in his support of adult stem cell therapy. "I tell people what it did for me and what it did for Nancy. It's all about awareness," Eddie says. "Once people become aware, the word has to get out. Now I understand why the doctors call it 'Stem Cell Revolution' – people need to be aware, so my job is to tell everybody I meet. Nobody gets past me: every time we meet somebody, we talk about stem cells – it's the topic of the night! Even at an art opening, I will talk about stem cells to anybody and everybody! There should be a channel on TV, 'Learn About Stem Cells,' and everybody who's ever had it done should go on there and brag about it. When I think about my asthma and how long I suffered with it – so many people are suffering, and they don't need to."

One of the many patients Eddie referred to us is his friend Sandy Smilovitz. Sometimes, a person's name offers a clue to their personality. Such is the case with Sandy: Talk with him for a few minutes and you'll soon be smiling; he could easily give a few professional comedians a run for their stand-up money. Sandy's sense of humor happens to be the gallows variety – because what he's usually joking about is his failing health. "When I turned 60, I did an inventory and discovered there wasn't a body part I had that worked," he says with a laugh. He's actually not kidding: Sandy is a type 2 diabetic with an ulcerated esophagus and a stomach hernia; he's had two surgeries on his arthritic right knee. What's more, he adds, "my kidneys are messed up; they don't function properly. That's a side effect of diabetes – it puts more pressure on your kidneys, and your kidneys eventually fail."

As if that weren't enough, Sandy is one of the 15 million Americans coping with COPD (chronic obstructive pulmonary disease), a disease of the lungs resulting in poor airflow that worsens over time. "I've always had breathing problems, ever since I was a kid," he explains. "I had bronchitis a lot. But it never really bothered me; it's only in the last five years that breathing became a real problem." If you've ever experienced severe shortness of breath, or a coughing episode that led to choking, watery eyes, and regurgitation, then multiply that by 20 and you'll be able to understand what COPD sufferers cope with every day. "I couldn't do anything," Sandy says. "It gets to a point where you can kind of fight through the pain and inability to breathe, but at some point you just have to sit down. A friend of mine does biofeedback, and he was teaching me how to breathe deeply – I'd have to sit and stop and relax and start thinking about breathing and get my breath right, so basically I couldn't do anything. I would have pain no matter what I did. Our driveway is about 100 feet long and it has about a seven degree grade, so it's steep-ish. Just walking up the driveway to get the mail made my lungs scream – there would be a clenching pain, as if somebody had their hands on my lungs and squeezed. So simple things like going to the market and walking around were pretty difficult. On top of that, you can have these panic attacks where you can't breathe – it's real difficult to overcome."

As the disease progresses, COPD patients must live with a nose tube attached to an oxygen tank that goes everywhere with them. "If it doesn't kill you, that's pretty much the bottom line for COPD," Sandy says. That is no joke. And yet, Sandy's funny bone was never compromised during his struggle with COPD. Describing his medical history, he sounds more like a seasoned Borscht Belt comic than the retired entrepreneur he is. When he first arrived at our office for a consultation, he was taking two oral medications and using an inhaler twice daily. His oxygenation level was between 82 and 84; normal is above 90. "I couldn't walk up the stairs in our house without having pain in my chest," he recalls. "I had a constant pain in the upper right quadrant of my lung, and I wheezed a lot. If my blood sugar got too high, my breathing got even worse." We treated Sandy for the first time in November 2012 (follow up treatment when?). "At our first consult, Dr. Lander said, 'I can't guarantee anything.' I said, if he could just stop the degeneration, however bad my lungs are I'll be happy. Dr. Lander did more than that; he corrected it. Within a week, I was walking up and down my driveway. I could breathe. I threw away the medication and the inhalers. My COPD has gone away completely; I don't have any breathing problems at all. I could probably run a marathon if it weren't for the fact that my knees, my feet, and my back are no good. But," he concludes with a well-timed smile, "at least I have my health!"

To hear Sandy describe it, his procedure was a great success. Today, he can walk down his hundred-foot driveway and get the mail, no problem. "Everything else is falling apart," he says with his signature laugh, "but when they put me into the ground, the only thing that'll be right is, I'll have great lungs. It's only because of the California Stem Cell Treatment Center. I truly believe it was miraculous; Dr. Lander saved my life. If I hadn't been treated with my stem cells, I would probably be on an oxygen bottle."

Chapter 5

STAYING IN THE GAME

Nobody wants to have "old guy problems" – not us, and certainly not our wives. So when patients come to us seeking relief from the physical symptoms of aging that eventually slow down everybody to some degree, we're excited about each new opportunity to investigate the applications of adult stem cell therapy. The reason is simple, and as personal as it is professional: We know that, in the not-too-distant future, those patients with old-guy problems could be us, and we want to do whatever we can to stay in the game, for our families and ourselves. We may make every effort to stay in shape, eat right, and adopt only healthy lifestyle choices; but old guy problems are like the relentless, resourceful stalker in the Blondie song "One Way or Another" who promises: *I'm gonna get ya, get ya, get ya.* Everyone has heard or spoken the phrase "age is just a number," most often repeated to palliate a person who's feeling insecure about his or her chronological years. But what if the chronology were reversed, and a person who's young in years – say, 38 years young – starts experiencing old guy problems? In such a case, that "palliative" phrase "age is just a number" carries absolutely no therapeutic effect.

Keith Warren (changed name as a last minute request to protect identity) played center for the several NFL teams before retiring. For those who don't know football, the center is a VIP of an MVP, the innermost position on a team's offensive line. The center's job is to pass the football to the quarterback by tossing it between his legs, in an exchange called "the snap" and then block someone nearly 300 pounds that's trying to tackle his quarterback. This happens at the start of each offensive play.

Years of snapping and blocking were bound to exert a great deal of repetitive stress on the center's hips. Even before retiring from the NFL in 2009, Keith was already feeling the effects of his unique occupational hazard, compounded when he sustained "a direct shock to the hip" that necessitated hip arthroscopy. Happily, keen intelligence is another occupational hazard of an NFL center, who has the best view of the defensive formation before the snap; he makes the first line call and may also be relied on for play-calling. Charged with so much responsibility, the center is the smartest player on the offensive line, and his career success depends less on brawn than on brains. Keith flexed the latter attribute when he began exploring treatment options for his hip pain, which by April 2013 had become excruciating. In football terminology, the player who receives the ball directly from the center is "under center" – and as fans of the game from way back, we were glad to be under center when Keith passed his hip problem to our office, choosing us to call the play. Incidentally, we have a special interest in helping athletes and former athletes overcome injuries sustained on the playing field, because we have our own in-house Division I football star: Mark's son Sean Berman who was a quarterback on the LA Tech roster, where he's was studying biology with the goal of becoming a doctor. Sean was ranked 47 by ESPN out of high school, in 2009. So, we reckon the day isn't far off that athletes and former athletes who consult CSCTC about treatment will be able to snap their problems to a physician with experience at play-calling both on the field and in the exam room: Dr. Berman the younger.

When Keith Warren stopped playing in 2009, the pressure to perform as a center was off. But staying in the game on everyday activities, even those us non-athletes take for granted, was beginning to prove more challenging than play-calling. By 2011, "I'd have pain walking up and down stairs, I'd have pain standing," Keith recalls, attributing his discomfort to "the physical challenges – no, the abuse – that my body took playing football." He was just 36 at the time. "The pain would shoot from my hip all the way down past my knee; I couldn't do a lot of stuff I wanted to do." Skiing, a favorite pastime, was now out of the question for Keith. But of all the activities he was now sidelined from, horsing around with his children was the one this Dad of four missed most. "I couldn't get down and play with my kids like I wanted to," he says. "I started noticing that I couldn't do most of the things I used to be able to do with them. My two older kids, twins, are real active in sports, so I try to help coach them. Then, it would just really start to ache while I was standing around in my job I do now." (Since retiring from the NFL, Keith has worked in orthopedic medical device sales.) "My clients are all orthopedic surgeons, so I would ask their opinion on what type of surgery I should have. They all agreed on a total hip replacement – but being in my mid-30s, I didn't feel like I was of age to get one of those operations." Then a sales colleague told Keith about CSCTC and our interest in using stem cell therapy to help pro athletes overcome debilitating pain due to occupational sports injury. He contacted us and, after a discussion and careful review of his medical records, we evaluated Keith to be eligible for treatment. But he didn't nail down a date until a few months later, by which time the pain could not be ignored. "I kind of put everything on hold and went down there [to Rancho Mirage]," Keith says.

Prior to treatment, "I tried every synthetic medication you could take; my hip was shot up probably 30 times because it hurt so bad," he recalls. After the first cortisone shot into Keith's hip, the pain was alleviated for almost three months; subsequent injections, however, proved less and less effective. "After a while, the cortisone would work for maybe a month and a half," he says. "Plus, it kills the circulation. Doctors say most people get four to six cortisone shots in a lifetime; I had more than that in a year." On the day of his treatment at CSCTC, in April 2013, our star center discovered what our fit and trim patients all commiserate about: a mini-liposuction is not for wimps, and the process of harvesting lipoaspirate from a person without much fat on him can result in significantly more soreness and bruising than a person with, say, a spare tire would feel. For this procedure to have the successful results we aim for, we needed the liposuction to yield at least one to five million cells per hip. "When I played, I was 300 pounds; now I weigh about 225, so that part was the worst," Keith admits. "I was pretty bruised up – my kids were impressed! – and I felt sore for a month and a half. Now, I'm in awe of people who go in and get a liposuction for cosmetic purposes." After we separated out Keith's stem cells in the centrifuge machine, the machine that tallies the viable cells – it's aptly named The Countess – let us know we succeeded in harvesting

121 million cells (a good percentage being stem cells, but technically including WBCs and other cells as well) from Keith's liposuction. We injected 44 million of those cells intravenously. Then, to ensure that the intra-joint injections would be absolutely precise, we moved him to our interventional radiology department for a CAT-scan-guided deployment of the remaining cells into his hips, under local anesthetic. Seventy-seven million of Keith's own cells were injected into his hips. As doctors, we're used to the "wow" factor of doing injections with sophisticated imaging, but Keith's not alone in remarking that, "It was phenomenal to see the needle go in under the scan – looking at X-rays is something I do anyway for my job, but this time I could see for myself when the doctors pointed out that I had bone spurs growing on the outside part of my hip."

When Keith left our office wearing an elastic-velcro binder around his waist to help reduce swelling, we told him that we estimated it would take between 24 and 48 hours for the initial anti-inflammatory properties of his cells to take effect on his damaged hip. He called to report that he first noticed positive effects within 24 hours. "After 48 hours, I felt like a million bucks," he says. "I got out of bed and it was like, oh my gosh, my hip has not felt this good for four years! And then, in the back of my mind, the skeptic in me was like, OK, this is just temporary. The doctors instructed me not to exercise or do anything for about eight days after the procedure, which is hard for me. My usual m.o. is, if someone says wait five days, I'll wait two; but I figured, for once I'm going to listen to the doctors. They also told me not to lift anything heavy; I'm like, OK, whatever... I did take off that elastic waist binder pretty quick! But this time, I waited the whole eight days and didn't do anything, not even ride the stationary bike. I took those eight days off, and afterward I felt great. Then I wished we'd done this [procedure] in January, when we first started talking about it. On the first day that I could perform physical activity, I said, all right, docs, let's see how it really worked – *I'm going to push this thing!* So I went on an eight-mile hike up this mountain. Eight days earlier, I literally could not walk, the pain was so debilitating. I ended up hiking and running that first week, maybe sixteen or 20 miles. Because I'd had so many shots that were just a temporary Band-Aid type of fix, I thought this might not last either, so I went a little overboard while I could. And it felt fine."

41

So, how do the cells actually work? This is a complex topic because it's not just the adult mesenchymal stem cells – it's the whole Stromal Vascular Fraction (SVF) with many kinds of cells bathed in cytokine growth factors (polypeptide signaling molecules). This "mother's soup" is superior to just cells alone. SVF has three main properties, and we try to use each to our benefit based on what we are trying to achieve clinically. The first property is "anti-inflammatory," which is effective for arthritis and other inflammatory diseases and can often be effective within 24-48 hours after treatment. Second is "regenerative" or "trophic effects," whereby the cells are capable of promoting healing by either directly replacing damaged cells or secreting cytokine growth factors that affect repair using cell-to-cell signaling. This effect takes weeks to months. The third is "immuno-modulatory," in which SVF mitigates auto-immune diseases by "re-booting" the immune system. Before any of these properties can occur, two important events must take place on a cellular level: the first critical aspect of SVF is that the stem cells must be attracted target tissue. This process is called "homing" in that the stem cells will preferentially travel to sites that secrete signaling molecules associated with damaged, inflamed, and degenerated tissue. The other essential event is that stem cells must be "activated" or "turned on" to effect healing by special triggers (other signaling molecules) as also associated with damage, disease, inflammation, or degeneration. The essence of the work we are doing at our treatment and research centers is to attempt to exploit any and all of these three main properties and 2 special events (homing and activation) to optimize clinical outcomes.

SIDEBAR – THE 3 PROPERTIES OF SVF after homing and activation

1. Anti-Inflammatory
2. Regenerative
3. Immuno-Modulatory ("re-boot the immune system")

In Keith's case, the first two properties were the main players in his treatment; SVF went to work simultaneously fighting inflammation in his damaged hips, and regenerating the connective tissue, i.e. cartilage, to cushion and promote ease of joint mobility. The third unit of the SVF army, the Immuno-Modulatory aspect, wasn't called for duty in this skirmish; however, the Homing and Activating forces did play a role, enabling the stem cells to locate the damaged areas of his body that needed an assist, and "turning on" his body's own healing power like an "On" switch, triggered by the inflammation and degeneration in his hips.

We checked in with Keith and reminded him that the cells wouldn't fully take effect until about three months after the injections – and that during that time, he'd have awesome days alternating with days when he didn't feel so hot, as his cells helped his body work to resolve the hip problem and self-heal. "The doctors were 100 percent right," Keith says. "I had great days and bad days – then at three months, it felt really, really good. That ache-y, shooting pain I used to have – I didn't have that pain any more, and I'm not taking any pain meds. I still have some pain in my hip, but it has nothing to do with what I was treated for; it's those bone spurs, because nothing could be done to change the structure of the bone. So the spurs hurt a bit, but other than that, I've got a range of motion in my hip that I haven't had in two years. I went back on the stationary bike, and started going for longer and longer runs; now I try to run at least two miles a day, taking Saturday off because the body needs rest. And we've been going on eight-to-twelve-mile hikes up Mammoth Mountain, where the elevation is about 10,000 feet. Before, I'd have to figure out how I was going to walk the next day after a workout, even with pain meds, which I no longer take. When I went skiing in February, I tell you, I was a mess for a week afterward. Now, I cannot wait to get back up on that mountain. I feel like I got it back." Here's what else he got back: healthy, competitive play time with his kids. Before his procedure, Keith was playing basketball with the 12-year-old twins and getting his butt kicked. "They'd never been able to beat me, but one day I wasn't feeling great, and they beat me," he remembers, adding with a grin: "We've played a couple of times since I had the procedure, and I smashed them! I had enough juice in my old legs to make sure they weren't going to beat me again."

Another one of our patients, Spencer Lehmann was 67 when he first came to CSCTC for a consultation; he gave us a pretty sobering description of what it's like trying to maintain one's normal routine on "old legs" – except his legs were the only part of this dynamic patient you could rightly classify as "old." It's one thing for a 38-year-old former NFL player in excellent shape to maintain a competitive edge on his teenage kids after just one cell treatment; now, how about an out-of-shape guy in his sixties getting a leg up on the 38-year-old? After extended time growing increasingly frustrated at being unable to do the activities one is used to doing, one inevitably puts on weight – that's a sad fact of life. But here's the good news: that unwanted belly fat, plus the occasional love handle, equals a rich reserve of adult stem cells that may be harvested more than once, for serial treatments that yield impressive results. Spence has 30 years on Keith, but he came through not one but three mini-liposuctions.

Although Spence was never a professional athlete, skiing was one of his passions – until back pain conspired with pain in his limbs to make moving down a mountain impossible. Infuriatingly, even walking became an activity as challenging as any giant slalom course. "One of my neighbors in Palm Springs, Nancy, had been overweight and walking with a cane for a while," he recalls. "You could tell that at one time she looked really good, but she'd been in a very bad car accident that smashed up her knees, and was up to nine Vicodins a day. Then, one day I noticed that Nancy had lost all her excess weight and didn't need her cane – she looked fantastic. So I asked her about her transformation, and she told me about CSCTC. This was in early 2012." At that point, Spence was actively resenting the braces he had to wear on his feet and ankles, to cope with the edema that would result from too much time spent on his feet. But the braces were a necessary evil; he'd been suffering from claudication of the calves due to narrowing arteries since 2009. "I couldn't walk a block without searing pain shooting down my calf," he says. "It was like somebody took a sharp knife, heated it in the oven, and ran it through my leg muscle."

Yet, like most of us, in his mind's eye Spence was still the young guy he remembered seeing in the mirror – the one who'd lifted weights since age 12, and started downhill skiing at 14, racing freestyle throughout high school and college; the one who still looked youthful when he hit forty. Spence continued skiing as usual, with a normal fighting weight of 160; but the pounds started piling on during his late forties as a result of chronic lower-back pain. A consultation with an orthopedist revealed that the last two discs in his spine had completely degenerated.

The orthopedist's verdict? "Either quit skiing, or be prepared to become paralyzed and never walk again," Spence recalls. "So I worked my ass off trying to make a success of my company." Spence also coped with problems in his first marriage that ultimately led to divorce, so his time got devoted to work, not workouts. "I started gaining an immense amount of weight, between sitting behind a desk and not being able to do the kind of exercise I wanted to do," he admits. "On top of the back pain, I also had severe arthritis in my knees; I was taking four salicylate pills check a day – 28 each month – and that's really tough on the kidneys."

His neighbor Nancy's success with cell therapy motivated Spence to call us and make an appointment. "The doctors said, 'You look tired and you're fat'," he recalls. "I mean, they said it much more politely than that, but I really appreciated their honesty. I thought, I like these guys already!" About a week later, on the first of June 2012, Spence underwent treatment at CSCTC. "During the liposuction, I said, while you're doing that, would you please take that extra 30 pounds out of there?" he remembers with a laugh. Fulfilling his request was impossible, of course; but the extra weight Spence was carrying enabled us to harvest much more than our minimum needed amount of material with ease – and that, in turn, let us address several of his issues in one treatment session. With Spence, we easily harvested two full syringes' worth (approximately 100cc) of fat in the same time as it took us to coax just one syringe of fat from young, buff Keith Warren. Guided by the CAT scan, our orthopedic radiology colleague Dr. John Feller, founder and chief of Desert Medical Imaging, injected 60 million of Spence's cells into his spine. As for the rest of the cell haul, "We got enough to give me injections in each calf for the claudication, a shot in each of my knees, and one in my left hip, for a problem I was having there too," Spence marvels. "I asked how long would it be before I'd feel any improvement; the doctors said I might start noticing something in about six weeks, but for sure in a couple of months. I'm a fiscal conservative," Spence adds with a laugh, "so it was only fitting that I got a conservative estimate!"

However, we were very happy to hear that Spence's cells spread their wealth quite liberally, imparting bodywide relief much more quickly than we could have hoped: he reported feeling substantial improvement upon waking up the morning after his treatment. "I got out of bed with no pain for the first time in years," he recalls. "I turned to my wife and said, 'I don't f***ing believe this!' She said, 'Maybe it's a fluke?' But I got up without pain the next day, and the day after that it was the same thing. After one week, I threw away those braces. Then, three weeks later we were in Las Vegas at the Wynn Hotel, which as you know is huge – figure at least half a mile from the tower to the meeting rooms, and probably longer – but I walked that distance to and from every day for a week with no pain in my calves, none."

"I feel better today, at 68, than I did when I was 50," Spence concludes. "What Mark Berman and Elliot Lander and that office did was give me back my life, in every sense of the word. And we're not through!" Spence is currently undergoing a series of stem-cell treatments for the oldest of old-guy problems in the book: erectile dysfunction. We'll keep you posted. As for his very kind words, it wasn't us – it was Spence's own cells doing their healing job. They certainly had strength in numbers: so many of Spence's problems are amenable to regenerative therapy, and the higher the cell count, the more effective the treatment appears to be, regardless of the patient's age.

Chapter 6

THE HARDER THEY COME

Few disorders are more devastating to think about or discuss – let alone experience – than Peyronies Disease, severe inflammation and scarring of the soft tissue of the penis. Just imagine the agony of guys who don't just think about, but also live with, this urologic disorder that affects more than 3% of men in the prime of their sexual life. Imagine if your penis – an organ that's normally the source of exquisite pleasure – were to suddenly cause terrible pain, both physical and psychological. Peyronies patients experience all the nightmare scenarios that could befall the penis: discomfort, shortening… loss of girth… abnormal curvature… indentation… erectile dysfunction. Peyronies has plagued men for hundreds of years – it got its name from the 18th century French surgeon Francois Gigot de la Peyronie – yet apart from a few promising pharmaceuticals, most mainstream remedies for it are decades, if not centuries, out-of-date. Some patients are offered surgical repair which often leads to more scarring, shortening or erectile dysfunction.

Patients have told us horror stories of physicians telling them to "just forget about sex – that part of your life is over." But sex, we believe, is an important barometer of overall well-being; it's not something to give up on without a fight. To those docs who tell their patients "There's nothing we can do," we say: "There's always something you can do." We feel the pain of Peyronies patients and their partners, so we were thrilled to discover that stem cell therapy can help these patients significantly, enabling them to regain a measure of their normal sexual function. Many cases of Peyronies are caused by trauma to the penis during intercourse, which results in scar tissue formation. Many cases occur for unknown causes and the condition can change spontaneously in curvature and severity until it enters a chronic phase in which scar is so hard it is occasionally calcified.

The full effect of Peyronies is evident when the penis is erect; while flaccid, it appears normal, but when engorged, it's curved. And the more scarring a penis has developed, the more hook-like it will be and eventually it can make penetration impossible in some cases... (Some beta blocker drugs list Peyronies as a possible side effect; targeting the beta receptors, this class of drugs is widely prescribed for the management of cardiac arrhythmias, hypertension, and protecting the heart from a second heart attack, but beta blockers are also frequently used by musicians, actors, and public speakers to combat performance anxiety and crippling stage fright.) When cases of Peyronies occur without any known cause, these are known as "idiopathic."

The body relies on adequate blood flow to bring stem cells to repair damaged tissue with minimal scar. As scar tissue builds up over time, it interferes with blood flow and erectile dysfunction results. Double ouch. Our patient Ryan had been feeling the pain and humiliation of Peyronies for four years prior to his diagnosis in 2008; added to that was his doctor's cold dismissal of Ryan's desire to find relief and resume sexual relations with Jane, his wife of 34 years. "At that time, I had a bunch of other stuff going on," Ryan recalls. "It was a dark period: I'd lost my job, I couldn't have sex, and my wife was threatening to leave me. I was telling this to my family practice doctor, who showed no sympathy at all. He was looking at his watch the entire time. 'I hope next year is better', he said, then ran out of the room!"

Happily for the couple, Ryan sought a second opinion, calling us in 2012 after an internet search led him to CSCTC. As his wife explains, "Coping with a disease like Peyronies helps you clarify and reconfirm your priorities, and the top priority for my husband and me was feeling healthy and young and vibrant." Their rate of marital relations had dwindled from two or three times a week to twice a year. "Almost more than the physical problems that prevented us from having intercourse, the hardest part was seeing the emotional damage being done to the man I love," Jane says. "It's terrible to see someone in such deep psychological pain – his pain was much worse than any disappointment that I might have had." The changes in the appearance of his penis were shocking and emasculating. As Ryan recalls, "I developed what's called an hourglass deformity, where the lower third of the shaft didn't fill out much during an erection, and that made it impossible to have penetration. It didn't work, and on top of that, I lost probably a third of the length that I had. I mean, it was terrible – one of those insult things." As psychologically emasculating as Peyronies is, the searing physical torture of it is nothing to sneeze at, especially during arousal. Here's how Ryan describes the painful lesions of scar tissue on his penis: "Like having a rock in your shoe when you're walking – when you get an erection, that's the sensation you have."

Before delivering his cells, we injected Ryan's penis with Lidocaine to numb the pain – but this process was slowed by the numerous lesions on his Tunica (the fibrous core structure of the penis) which were so scarred that, in several places, we couldn't insert the needle. Many of the lesions were on the base of the shaft, which we wanted to target with Ryan's stem cells, so the painkilling process turned into somewhat of a killer. Stromal Vascular fraction was the injected directly into the plaque (?using multiple penetrations with the deployment needle). After it was all over, we warned Ryan not to freak out when, in a few hours' time, his penis would look like someone had hit it with a hammer. "It was pretty swollen and completely black," Ryan remembers. "I took Tylenol for the pain, but I didn't stay sore for long." It was several weeks before he noticed an improvement. Then, about four months later, after his second of three treatments, "I got the length back," he says, "and those hard lumps of scar tissue started sort of dissolving away. I still have part of the hourglass, but it's a lot better than it was; I got most of my girth back." Today, he reports, "The penis doesn't bend like it did, and my stability – meaning my ability to keep an erection – is completely improved. I'm able to put it in my wife and keep it there. That's the beauty of the stem cell thing: after three treatments, I got it all back."

His penis, Ryan adds, is "pretty close to what it used to be. One side is more caved in than the other; I notice it, but my wife says it's no big deal. I'm very happy." So is Jane: "Even when things are at their worst, there are creative things you can do to be intimate without penetration," she says, "but having a husband who's feeling confident and better about himself is a turn-on." Today, Ryan is satisfied with his new job and his healthy sex life. As for the frequency, Jane adds, "Maybe it's not every day, but there's certainly a lot of intimacy." Perhaps most sexy of all is the courage Ryan displayed in refusing to let his quality of life be compromised by a condition that his doctors had told him just could not be helped. "I really admire my husband's courage for going out on a limb," Jane concludes. "He didn't know anyone who'd already had this type of treatment, so it seemed pretty experimental at the time. But instead of feeling humiliated, he went with it."

Ryan's success helped us learn a lot about Peyronies disease. His outcomes data was included in our original series of five patients who all had spectacular results and were presented at the Western Section American Urologic Association in November, 2013 and at the American Association of cosmetic Surgeons Annual Meeting in January of 2015. We have gone on to treat many more cases of Peyronies and have improved therapy by adding a series of low intensity shock wave treatments to the Peyronies tissue to help stem cells home and activate to optimize healing.

###

Chapter 7

WALK ON

Muscular Dystrophy (MD) is a group of nine inherited, progressive muscle diseases. All forms of MD cause muscle weakness and muscle loss. Some forms – notably, Duchenne MD – appear in early childhood, while others don't emerge until middle age, and sometimes even later. Even within each type of MD, doctors see variations in terms of the muscles affected and the symptoms experienced by individual patients. Some people have mild cases that worsen slowly; severe cases, on the other hand, are disabling. But there is one thing all forms of MD have in common: All worsen as the patient's muscles grow weaker, and most people with MD end up unable to walk. According to virtually every authority on the subject, there is no cure for MD; the standard medical wisdom tells patients and their families that symptoms may be helped by treatments such as physical and speech therapy, as well as orthopedic devices, surgery, and medications.

MD has become almost as politically charged as the topic of stem cells. For forty-four years, this disease's claim to fame was the Muscular Dystrophy Association of America's long-running annual Labor Day telethon hosted by actor-comedian Jerry Lewis. Celebrities ranging from Joan Crawford to John Lennon and Yoko Ono made appearances, urging TV viewers to donate money to the cause, which collected more than two billion dollars. But the telethon came under fire in recent years for using disabled people in wheelchairs – particularly children – as fundraising tools. "Jerry's Kids," as the telethon called them, were portrayed as objects of pity, while Lewis made maudlin appeals to the television audience, promising "we're closer than ever to a cure." Critics assert that emphasizing cures to "normalize" people with disabilities detracts from efforts to provide them with basic civil rights, such as employment opportunities and accessible transportation and housing. They argue that Jerry Lewis merely preached pity for people with MD, when what they really deserve is respect. (The Muscular Dystrophy Association phased out the telethon, and Lewis as its spokesperson, replacing it in 2012 with an annual Labor Day TV event called "The MDA Show of Strength.")

Each year that he hosted the telethon, Lewis performed the MDA signature song "You'll Never Walk Alone" from the Rodgers and Hammerstein musical "Carousel." Its lyrics go like this:

> *When you walk through a storm hold your head up high and don't be afraid of the dark*
> *At the end of the storm is a golden sky and the sweet silver song of a lark*
> *Walk on through the wind, walk on through the rain, though your dreams be tossed and blown*
> *Walk on; walk on, with hope in your heart and you'll never walk alone*

Disability rights activist Mike Ervin, the most outspoken critic of the "Jerry's Kids" pity-the-patient culture is himself a former telethon poster child who once appeared on TV with Lewis. Renowned in the blogosphere as "Smart Ass Cripple" (also the title of his blog), the wheelchair-bound Ervin has many fans, among them the late film critic Roger Ebert, who likened him to "a standup comedian who can't stand up." Ervin is the subject of the 2005 documentary "The Kids Are All Right," in which he and other MD patients style themselves as "Jerry's Orphans." With all due respect to Ervin and many other vocal critics of the Jerry Lewis approach, is it wrong for people with MD to hold out hope for a cure? We don't think so.

Whether or not it's politically correct, many did continue to hope – but perhaps none more fervently than Regina Chauvin. "I always believed they'd find a cure, hopefully in my lifetime," affirms the Louisiana native. She is not one of "Jerry's Kids," nor is she one of "Jerry's Orphans." She's a person who was diagnosed with Limb-Girdle Muscular Dystrophy

(LGMD) and, although wheelchair-bound, remained determined that one day she would enjoy life without the debilitating effects of this disease. "I was born with nothing wrong, and I grew to be a normally active child, dancing ballet and tap, and playing sports," remembers Regina, now 33. "I loved all outdoor activities, especially softball, basketball, and track." Then, when she reached the age of thirteen, her heel cords – the Achilles tendon – started contracting. "I was walking on my tiptoes," Regina recalls. That's when she was diagnosed with Limb-Girdle Muscular Dystrophy. My condition kept declining, and by the time I was fifteen, I was using the wall to help myself walk – I had no balance, I was losing muscle mass and strength. By the age of 29, it was hard for me to walk even while holding somebody's hand, so I started relying on a power chair more and more." Regina resolved that she would – in the words of the old MDA song – walk on.

Without pleading for pity, it's fair to say that quality of life for MD patients is often very negatively impacted by the disease. Although a beautiful, vibrant young woman, Regina felt self-conscious about dating. With LGMD, it becomes increasingly difficult to lift the front part of the foot, and this causes one to trip. Regina often worried what would happen if she were out on a date and "might have to go to the bathroom, but wouldn't be able to stand up and walk – or would trip and fall!" For what she fully believed would be the day doctors would find a cure for MD, Regina bravely prepared herself like a dedicated athlete gearing up to compete in an Ironman Triathlon. Regina contacted us after she heard about another woman in her home town in Louisiana who had a successful treatment at our center for interstitial cystitis which is a very painful bladder condition that has no effective treatments and is known to make people feel like they have a urinary infection that "never goes away.". The first thing we explained to Regina is that we really cannot talk in terms of cure, since we don't currently have the technology to cure her condition. However, we did relay to her that we had treated several MD patients with excellent results in terms of mitigating their muscle damage and stiffness. We explained to her that she may be able to achieve similar results, with the possibility that she may require multiple treatments over a period of years, and soon we may be able to freeze her cells through our "Cells On Ice" program, allowing recurrent administration which are vital in degenerative conditions like Muscular Dystrophy.

We treated Regina on August 6, 2014. "I had the procedure in Rancho on a Wednesday, and was back home on Friday. I didn't notice any changes immediately," she adds, "although I entered the clinic in a push chair, and right after my cells were injected, I remember walking out of the treatment room with assistance from the nurse. I was really tired, maybe because of traveling from Louisiana to California. I think I slept sixteen hours straight in California! The next day after coming home, Saturday morning, I felt some of my muscles getting stronger. I felt it first in my legs: they were starting to work again." Before, the simplest tasks so many of us take for granted were major hurdles in Regina's average day. "If I was sitting in a chair and wanted to grab a piece of clothing, or a towel on the floor, I would have had a really hard time coming back up to the sitting position, much less carrying that towel with me," she says. "Now I can do it in four motions, rather than trying to jerk myself everywhere."

In October, Regina called our office to report a dramatic improvement: "I feel like about 95 percent of my muscles are working again – it almost feels like I have the muscles of a newborn baby! Now I've just got to build and strengthen the muscle. I still use the wheelchair when nobody is here to help me; but I get on my feet and walk around the house and do things I couldn't do before." Imagine laundry not as a dreaded chore, but an activity you'd be more than happy to do – if only you had the strength to load the washer, then empty it and place its contents in the dryer. "Another thing I can do now is laundry," Regina reports. "I wash my bed sheets, take them out of washer, and put them in dryer. Before, just bending down and getting laundry out of the machine was a challenge – I couldn't even open the dryer! And I can just about dress myself; I still need help with jeans or anything that's kind of tight. But for the most part, I can put on my own bra and shirt."

That's not all that's improved. "I walk straighter now – I don't have as much of a sway in my gait as I did before, because I don't have to jerk myself to give me that extra push." What's more, the symptom that first marked the onset of her MD – tightened heel cords – showed major signs of improvement. "My heel cords started out with the right one at negative 48 and the left at negative 38. As of my last Active Release session, the right one measured negative 20 and the left negative

5 – that's very significant. I can also walk better without shoes; before I couldn't, because I had no balance." Some of our fashion-conscious patients with orthopedic issues complain that they cannot wear their beloved heels, and many are thrilled to be able to return to gravity-defying footwear post-stem cell therapy (including Mark's wife Saralee, who has quite a collection of stilettos). Regina was the opposite: She longed to wear flats, but needed the support that a heel provided. "Because of the contraction in my Achilles tendon, I couldn't wear a shoe without a heel, because my heels didn't touch the ground," she explains. "Now I switch between my favorite pair of flip-flops and my tennis shoes – which I couldn't wear for the past four years!"

Regina has a strong character; that inner fortitude reveals itself in her physical endurance and high tolerance of pain. Her commitment to exercise would be an integral part of her success. Immediately after treatment, we had her see Michael Butler, an elite trainer and expert in active release techniques in Palm Desert, California, and he started Regina on an aggressive regimen of physical therapy. Active release is a movement based massage technique that treats problems with muscles, tendons, ligaments, fascia, and nerves. It works by relieving tension throughout the body's muscles and fibrous tissues. This therapy is not for the faint of heart. Whereas traditional massage is relaxing, deep muscle therapy can be quite uncomfortable and even painful at times, as the practitioner must apply more pressure in order to stimulate the deeper muscles and tissues surrounding them. Regina continued her physical therapy religiously once she returned to Louisiana. "It was excruciatingly painful, to the point where I could have cried," says Regina, who resolutely pushed through the pain. Her dedication to twice-weekly Active Release sessions is a clear indication of her determination to beat MD. In addition, Regina set aside two days of each week for physical and occupational therapy. She was impressively diligent about complying with all of our advice, and her extraordinary motivation contributed to her positive results.

Before going to bed, Regina downs a protein shake, a mix of whey and time-release casein, "so that while I'm sleeping my muscles are well fed." Prior to working out, she takes C4, a powdered nutritional supplement favored by bodybuilders (its active ingredient is creatine). She also takes several supplements for optimum cellular health, including vitamin D3, nitric oxide, and L-Arginine. Many of our patients take nitric oxide after their procedures, since it improves vascularity and blood flow, and has been shown to help stem cells differentiate. It is a simple remedy made of beets and hawthorn; Neo40 makes the best quality nitric oxide that actually provides you with the enzyme your body needs to turn nitrates into nitric oxide. (On a side note, we were surprised when Regina told us of her scientific interest in cannabis, and that she smokes marijuana every day as an adjunct therapy. Wherever you stand on the controversial topic of medical marijuana, Regina's positive results offer anecdotal evidence that cannabis doesn't seem to interfere with stem cells' ability to differentiate.)

Her avid interest in a healthy diet and exercise routine is partly the influence of her boyfriend, a bodybuilder. "I started dating him earlier this year, even before I found out about stem cell therapy," Regina says. "He's the one that really got me on those supplements, and he helps with my workouts too. He's been a big supporter, always encouraging and motivating me." Like so many people with degenerative diseases such as MD, Regina hadn't previously been so lucky in love. "Every day, I felt like I had less of a chance of finding somebody who'd be patient and want to help," she admits. "I had several good relationships, but nobody could ever commit. The fear of what might happen to me, would my condition get worse, and how would they take care of me – I think all this was in the back of their minds, plus my not being able to work a full-time job, and the pressure of having to support a disabled person. That hurt my previous relationships."

Since her treatment, Regina has been walking tall in many aspects of her life, professionally as well as personally. "With every day that I make progress, I feel closer to seeing my dreams become reality," she says. "I found the right guy, I think I have the right connections to find the perfect job… I can see everything falling into place. I think it's amazing that I could have this opportunity to feel this way. I'm so thankful I was able to get the treatment, because otherwise I would be steadily getting worse." She feels ready to seek full-time employment again. "I have a couple different job opportunities," Regina says. Although she's trained as a tax preparer, her experience with stem cells – and her sincere wish to help raise awareness so that more patients might be helped – is encouraging her to explore politics as a possible future career path. As part of her new calling for public service, Regina started the Facebook group "Stem Cell Therapy – Why Is It Not FDA Approved?" and posts regularly about her progress.

As a teenager, Regina "did a lot of running, but I haven't been able to run since I was fifteen years old – and that was eighteen years ago. I want to run again." She eagerly anticipates the day her running shoes will see serious action for the first time since her high-speed, high school days. When she can finally strap them on, stretch her legs, and let rip, where would Regina like to go? "Wherever my feet will take me." In the meantime, she's warming up for that milestone run – with weight training – and putting on her own show of strength for the delight of her friends and family. "Before, gravity was enough weight resistance, but now I'm actually able to work out with weights attached to my legs and arms," she concludes. "I'm building muscle – and that's something doctors had always told me was impossible with MD."

Chapter 8

VISION QUEST

As practicing MDs with a combined fifty years of experience, we are acutely aware of the need for prescription medications. We would never argue, as some of our detractors suggest, that stem cells could ever replace doctor-prescribed pharmaceuticals. However, there are cases in which prescription meds simply cannot be a long-term answer for certain patients – cases for which stem cells offer a life-changing alternative to drugs that, taken over an extended period of time, carry more risks than benefits. One of these medications is Prednisone, in the category of corticosteroids. These synthetic drugs are widely prescribed because they work extremely well as immune-suppressants – i.e. they slow down the immune system when it becomes abnormally overactive, as in cases of autoimmune disease (when the body literally attacks itself), or organ transplant, or cancer. But the limitations of corticosteroids – and the urgent need for a therapeutic alternative – became dramatically apparent when ophthalmologist Larry Geisse, MD contacted us about one of his patients in 2011.

One year earlier, in November 2010, Julia Matsumoto went to see Dr. Geisse, complaining of sudden vision loss. The 31-year-old was a fit, active wife and mom of two who had had no prior health problems. But, after what she describes as "a severe headache," Julia began experiencing substantial vision loss. The world looked "darker and darker," she recalls, and within a month, her field of vision was reduced to "the size of a pin-drop, and eventually, complete darkness." The diagnosis was optic neuritis, an autoimmune swelling of the nerve connecting the brain to the eyes. It's not known what causes optic neuritis, but by all accounts, the gradual vision loss that results is terrifying. The term "gradual" is relative, and individual to each case: Some patients experience optic neuritis in one eye, and it takes just a few hours for the vision in that eye to darken; then, inexplicably, the vision might return later. Other patients experience optic neuritis in both eyes, and it takes a period of weeks before their diminishing sight is almost entirely gone.

"She has an autoimmune optic neuritis, or perhaps Chronic Relapsing Inflammatory Optic Neuropathy, we're not really sure which," Dr. Geisse explains. "Typical optic neuritis, as with MS, is rapid in onset, but usually recovers over time with treatment, and usually [involves] one episode, or another episode years later. This type of optic neuritis, on the other hand, runs a progressive, downhill course with no recovery, with each episode resulting in further loss of vision that is not recoverable. This occurs over a very short time, and is usually somewhat responsive to very high doses of steroids." The cause of this condition is unknown. "For some reason, her body was attacking itself, causing inflammation and damaging the optic nerve," Dr. Geisse says. "No one knows why it happens." What doctors do know is that corticosteroids have proven effective at slowing vision loss in optic neuritis cases. So, Dr. Geisse prescribed Prednisone to manage Julia's optic neuritis and prevent further vision loss. The dosage she needed to prevent further vision loss was 100 milligrams per day in addition to weekly intravenous delivery of methylprednisolone (Solu-Medrol).

But that RX came with an extreme adverse effect. After three months on the medication, Julia's quality of life suffered significantly. The steroids caused her to experience dramatic weight gain; within three months, she was 100 pounds overweight and morbidly obese. "I was working out five days a week – I used to take spin class, do weight lifting and crunches, go running – but with the Prednisone, it was as if someone put a tire pressure monitor on me: I was literally just blowing up," Julia says. "It was ridiculous. I wouldn't even be eating – that was the scary part. At one point," she adds, "my skin became so brittle that I couldn't tolerate underwear; I had to wear a muumuu. I was bleeding; I would take a shower, and my skin would melt off." There were stretch marks on Julia's arms, because her skin – unable to cover her rapidly expanding body mass – was stretched to the breaking point. The combination of weight gain and vision loss resulted in an inability to exercise. Another side effect of Prednisone is severe joint pain, which Julia felt with every movement. While her body would not stop expanding, her bones were becoming dangerously thinner, weaker, and more fragile – another adverse effect of long-term steroids that results in osteoporosis, which makes exercise risky due to the increased likelihood of fracturing. Julia's mostly sedentary existence was a terrible contrast to the life she used to know. "It got to a point where I couldn't walk, I couldn't enjoy my life," she says, her eyes welling with tears at the painful memory. "I was slowly dying from the medication." But without the high steroid doses, her vision rapidly vanished.

Her ophthalmologist agreed: "She was hardly recognizable," recalls Dr. Geisse. "Her skin was stretched so tight that it was splitting in areas. She could hardly move her joints. She had tremendous joint pain and back pain; she was very weak and could not walk. Her stomach hurt all the time despite the use of Proton Pump Inhibitors to protect the stomach. She was sick all the time with colds, since the Prednisone was suppressing her immune system. Her bones became very thin." Together, Julia and her doctor had to confront a wrenching dilemma. In Dr. Geisse's words, "Is it better to let a patient go blind than to kill her with steroids? Basically, to save her life, we had to stop the medication – even if it meant going blind. She had come to that point."

Julia was slowly weaned off the steroids. "It was very difficult to do, because I knew I would lose my sight," she says, "but it was the only choice for me at the time. I told my daughter that I would always remember the way she looked, so she'd have to describe to me her prom dress, her wedding dress…" When she lost her vision, Julia also lost her job and her medical coverage. Under the weight of that triple setback, she began the difficult process of recovering mobility with the long, white cane that visually impaired people use to detect objects in their path. "That was very hurtful and frustrating," she remembers. "I literally was running into everything. I would constantly hit the kitchen counter with my hip in the same spot – I could never learn that stupid corner, and it would make me so mad I cannot even express it! I would count the steps, but I'd still bang into it every single time, resulting in the worst bruising." The steroid medications also interfered with Julia's sleep: "I'd have to lie down because I'd be lucky if I could get two hours of sleep a day."

Dr. Geisse envisioned a happier ending to Julia's story, so he began researching alternatives to help her. "She's just the kind of person that touches your heart," he says. "The feeling you have is that you would do anything to get her better." The doctor began investigating stem cell therapy. "When I called the fifteen or so treatment centers in the U.S., Canada, and Mexico, each one of them had a sales person call me to discuss the treatment protocol and then try and sign Julia up," Dr. Geisse recalls. "Only Dr. Berman and Dr. Lander called me back as physicians to discuss the case, and only they said that there was a small chance this might help her, and that they had not treated anyone for this problem before. The other centers all said Julia would respond well with the treatment and virtually guaranteed that she would be cured – that was obviously a sales pitch. I appreciated these doctors' honesty, and the fact that this center seemed to be really trying to help patients and not just make money. So, we went with them."

We were eager to find out how Julia's condition would respond to treatment with her own cells, so we scheduled an appointment for her at our Beverly Hills location. We then learned that Julia's worsening condition had resulted in the loss of her job and her health coverage, and that her husband had also lost his job. "No money, no insurance, no doctors to help; the health care system abandoned Julia to go blind in her time of crisis," Dr. Geisse says, "and [her insurance carrier] just booted her out the door when she could not pay for their services." So we agreed to treat Julia at no cost. Mark gave Julia her first treatment in November 2011. Julia remembers thinking, "I don't have anything else to lose." But none of us – not Julia, her ophthalmologist, nor any of us at CSCTC – could have predicted the tremendous gains that started accruing after that initial treatment.

"I saw her a few days after the procedure, and I'm telling you, it was just miraculous," Dr. Geisse says. "With the stem cells, we can keep her vision and keep her off the steroids completely – that just in itself has been like a miracle." Thus far, Julia has lost 70 pounds. If you've ever seen a hummingbird in motion, then you know it's not always possible to see the color markings on these tiny, fast-moving flyers even if one has no visual impairment. "We have a dwarf citrus tree in our back yard," Julia explains, "and I was sitting outside, when suddenly something jumped off a tree branch and whizzed by me," Julia recalls. "All I noticed was something red – but I hadn't been able to see color for such a long time. So I asked my husband, 'What was that red thing?' 'That's a hummingbird,' he said." The red she saw was the bird's crimson plumage – she'd identified the color correctly. Her response? "That's the most beautiful thing I've ever seen – and then I just bawled."

Today, Julia sees different stripes and colors – notably, the ones marking the traffic lanes and signs near her home. Seven months after folding up her white cane, Julia passed her driver's test with her current vision, and is able to operate her vehicle to access the shopping mall across the street from where she lives. "It's nothing compared to how it was when I used to drive," she's quick to add. "The mall is literally right across the street, about 100 feet away." We think she's being modest; that's a huge driving distance for someone who, three years earlier, had resigned herself to a life without sight.

As doctors applying stem cells to vision loss, we still have a long road ahead of us. It would be wonderful if we could completely cure Julia's problem. We doubt that we are curing it, but we are definitely reversing it, and maybe stabilizing it. Part of the challenge is that her condition may be a variant of MS, and there is a circle of thought that suggests you need to knock out the autoimmune cells that are attacking the optic nerve, and then restore the nerve function with the SVF. Actually, there are some MS studies in which the SVF first attacks the autoimmune cells to wipe them out before trying to repair the damage with fresh stem cells. This may indeed become the chosen protocol, but for right now, we're getting some positive responses from SVF alone. As we progress, we'll figure out optimal treatment protocols.

Julia is one of our most gratifying success stories, and we've decided to keep treating her as long as she needs us to. Mark saw the ultimate validation of that decision when he received a holiday greeting that he calls, "Probably one of the most heartwarming Christmas cards I ever received in my life." It was a hand-drawn and –lettered note from Julia's daughter that read: "Thank You for giving my Mom a second chance. Now she can watch me drive ... play sports ... grow up ... graduate." Mark has treated Julia every two months since her first procedure. Yes, that is a lot of liposuctions, but in Julia's case, she'd gained so much weight from the steroids that she not only produces more fat, but also more stem cells. Our future plans to cryo-preserve cells through our "Cells On Ice" program will enable patients like Julia to have multiple stem cell deployments at far less cost and far greater convenience. At one recent treatment, we harvested 80 million viable cells. Because the local anesthesia, when done well, is nearly painless, the liposuction is painless and the only pain is the discomfort around the liposuction site as it's healing. She's quite a trooper to endure this; however, it is easier than going to the dentist (at least, that's what our patients generally tell us). "It's so difficult to explain," Julia concludes. "It's like I've done everything else, and then I did this, and my own body is healing itself."

*

Often, when people spot someone with a visual disability, the first instinct is to want to grab the person's hand or arm and help guide them. Julia Matsumoto certainly experienced her share of this. But, although Chad Rivera has what he calls "a little bit of a vision issue" – he is, in fact, legally blind – he rarely elicits that type of response. And he's fine with that. A natural athlete all his life, he's been an avid skateboarder since age four. These days, he not only skateboards, he also snowboards and exercises his passion for the martial arts – both activities that he undertook for the first time, amazingly enough, *after* his vision became impaired.

If you happen to be out snowboarding, it's easy to spot Chad: he'll be the one with his goggles hanging rakishly off the back of his helmet, "because they obstruct my vision." You might also spy him running confidently alongside vehicular traffic in shorts and flip-flops, on his way to an appointment. Watching him in motion, your first instinct is admiration, not pity. Looking much younger than his 47 years, Chad makes you think of a Japanese anime character, or perhaps one of the

X-men, come to life – especially when he's practicing jiu jitsu while wearing his signature, super-cool Moya Brand gi (the kimono-style apparel worn by martial artists). He gets around town on foot or on his bicycle, "with music in one ear and my traffic ear open." When riding his bike, Chad explains, "rather than waiting for the light, I'll go with the flow of traffic. I only take calculated risks, after analyzing the situation. That's how I've been wired, since way before I lost my eyesight."

But even when he's not navigating traffic on his bike, or surfing at upwards of 20 mph around a high-walled skate park, or perfecting his jiu jitsu moves, Chad simply does not move through life like someone who cannot see. There's nothing tentative or cautious about this guy. During a conversation, it's easy to forget he's blind because he makes convincing eye contact. He also responds more quickly to texts than many people we know who have no visual impairment! In fact, his "disability" only reveals itself to bystanders in certain circumstances: say, when his wife Tiffany parks in a space reserved for people with disabilities. Hopping out of their car, both looking fit and active, Chad and Tiffany are frequently confronted by other motorists chiding them for their choice of parking spot! "I'm pretty fortunate to have a sense of humor, so I'll just crack a joke," Chad says. "Just because someone's disability isn't flashed out there…" he adds, smiling and shaking his head.

Chad's impressive adjustment to such a devastating physical setback is due partly to the fact that he wasn't born blind. "For the first 22 years of my life, I could see," he points out. "You'd be surprised at what you can do when you have a memory of sight, even 25 years later. My world is still very colorful." In 1989, at age 22, Chad was completing college, studying art and graphic design and gaining a following for his "very intricate ink drawings," done with a .18 millimeter pen, "so the ink comes out the size of a hair." "I started as an agriculture major, but I always had a passion for art, so I ended up going to Laguna Beach Art School," he recalls. He went to work for his father, who grew grapes in the Coachella Valley, and soon after that, met the love of his life, Tiffany. Then, within a year, he started experiencing cloudy vision in one of his eyes. "I was like, whatever – maybe I stayed out too late the night before," Chad recalls. "I'd rub my eye and the cloudiness would go away." Then, one day Chad went to pick up his mother with his car. "At the second stop light after leaving the lot, it hit me," he remembers. "My vision went all cloudy and blurry, and I couldn't see the stop light. Rubbing the eye did nothing. I had to pull over and let my Mom drive."

The diagnosis: Leber's Hereditary Optic Neuropathy (LHON). This degeneration of the retinal ganglion cells and their axons leads to acute or sub acute loss of central vision. LHON affects mainly young adult males, and it's mitochondrially inherited – i.e., transmitted from mother to child (men cannot pass the disease to their kids). The toughest part for Chad – after learning that his mystery ailment was permanent, not lens-corrective, and not responsive to any medication – was getting used to seeing the world as if "looking through a foggy shower door." When all that sank in, he went through a long and very difficult adjustment period. "It was a good ten years of anger that made me passively suicidal – I didn't really give a crap anymore," Chad admits. "I was always the good-time guy, the one that would pick up and go on the spur of the moment – now, suddenly I'm imprisoned? I can't pick up and go anymore? I tried to push Tiffany away because I figured, at this point, I was defective. Thankfully, as hard as I tried to push her away, she saw enough in me to stick around, and we ended up developing a more serious relationship, then getting married."

Chad gave up drawing. "The passion wasn't there anymore," he says. For a while, he also gave up skateboarding, the sport he'd always loved. But helping raise his two sons – including changing diapers himself, swiftly administering CPR when one of the boys almost choked on a piece of candy, and, later, experiencing their first baby skateboarding steps – motivated Chad to get back on a skateboard, with his boys' enthusiastic encouragement. Now, it's hard to imagine him *not* bowl-riding. One thing Chad never gave up was the hope that his vision might improve. His philosophy is, "Don't be afraid to try," so he followed every possible therapeutic lead, however bogus-sounding – and as doctors, we confess that some of the snake-oil "remedies" he tried had us shaking our heads. "I've always been a take-chances type of person," Chad explains, in his typical bring-it style, "so I tried everything from antioxidant supplements to cayenne pepper drops prescribed by a Cuban faith healer. One year, I traveled to Tijuana every three weeks with a pocket full of cash, for shark-cartilage injections in my hip!"

The life-changer for Chad was his active pursuit of the martial arts, which he began at his wife's suggestion. Today, he holds a brown belt in judo *and* jiu jitsu. As he improved his moves, he also adopted a healthier lifestyle, juicing his share of carrots and spinach. "I figured as long as I stay healthy, maybe one day I'll get the opportunity to improve my sight," he says. The chance to treat Chad with his own stem cells, and to find out how a condition like his would respond, was an even bigger opportunity for us. The prevalence rate of LHON is approximately one in 30,000 people in the United States. But finding a patient with Chad's indefatigably positive outlook is even rarer still. Chad was referred to us in 2013 by one of our MD colleagues at Eisenhower Medical Center in Rancho Mirage, California (where Elliot has been on staff for seventeen years and served as past Chief of Urology). We treated Chad in March 2013. After we extracted fat from Chad's lower back, his cells were deployed intravenously; we could not inject the cells directly into his eyes, because at that time we were still awaiting approval from our IRB Institutional Review Board to perform intra-ocular injections.

There's not a lot of fat on Chad because he's in such great physical shape, so we had to work to extract what fatty tissue he did have. Still, we managed to harvest an impressive number of cells at Chad's first liposuction: 130 million. Lean patients sometimes end up having a greater number of more viable cells than those with, say, a spare tire. That's because the cells haven't been committed to forming fat, so they're actually available as primitive cells, a.k.a. pre-adipocytes, which have very potent regenerative properties. When we first started treating patients with their own fat-derived cells, we thought heavier people would have the advantage of more cells, but that was a misconception. With leaner patients, most of the cells come in the form of these potent pre-adipocytes, which helps us get a good result.

But at the end of the day, only our patients can tell us how good the result really is. Here's Chad's assessment after two treatments, during which his cells were injected intravenously: "My vision is still poor, but I did notice a little bit of change: colors definitely appear richer now. Within a couple of weeks after that first treatment, walking down the street, I'd notice that things almost looked like they were wet, because the color was popping out more. I've also gained a bit of depth perception, and although it's very slight, it definitely helps my skateboarding." Chad's perception of color and depth isn't all that's deepened. So has his insight into being blind. "It's been more than half of my life, its part of who I am," he says. "So now, I try to have fun with it. I'll be the first to crack a joke about it. I still have my moments, but every day is healing, so as time goes on, I'm dealing with it better." Had he not become blind, he might never have been set on his current athletic path: Working toward his black belt in the martial arts. "That helped repair me mentally," he says. "It's one of the most positive things that entered my life since LHON first came on – apart from my family, of course."

We're eager to inject Chad's cells directly into his eyes; our goal is for the direct injection to assist his cells in locating their target, resulting in even more vision improvement. A goal we can now attain since we have IRB approval for eye injections since October 2014. Chad returned for a second liposuction and IV injection in September 2013. We were so glad to see that he needed no help walking down the hall of our office; he was also identifying colors better. His extreme-athletic lifestyle can be rough on the extremities, so we were happy to hear that his follow-up treatment had some very positive side effects, even if these didn't relate to his vision:

"Physically, I felt my overall stamina was back on the map," Chad says. "I felt good, stimulated, like I just drank coffee. Training with professional athletes in their early 20s, I was able to keep up. Some repetitive-stress injuries throughout my body were kind of disappearing too. I felt rejuvenated – especially my feet, which are always in pain because of all the physical activity I do, and because I don't wear supportive shoes. One foot had been hurting really bad – but then, after the second treatment, both feet felt better." He's convinced his treatment helped his skating by alleviating repetitive-stress discomfort in his joints – and for Chad, that's a major quality of life issue because, as he will tell you, "If I can't skate anymore, I'm done."

As for his vision after that second treatment, Chad told us he could see the edge of the skate bowl's coping better while concrete surfing, and that his peripheral vision had improved slightly. "Of course I want to get cured," he says, "but if I end up helping other LHON patients, I'll be just as happy to open up that door of opportunity. My style is to leave no stone unturned; I'm never afraid to take that turn down that dark path. I'll be the first to go check out something new." Although he's given up drawing, Chad continues to express himself creatively through a different medium: "I make videos and I do all my own editing," he says. As he commented recently on Facebook, "I just point and shoot. I'm bound to capture something." With the help of a Zacuto Z-Finder attached to his Canon 7D camera, Chad now confidently captures still images as well as videos, and posts them on his Instagram feed (@ chadrivera). "I know what I'm shooting," he explains, "but I can't tell what I'm shooting until I get home and magnify the image," which he does using a projector-magnifier on his computer. That's when he sees the big picture: "The world," Chad concludes, "is still a great place."

Chapter 9

GO WITH YOUR GUT

When we opened the California Stem Cell Treatment Center, we made a conscious decision not to advertise our new practice. Our reasoning was that we were doing investigational work and if we were successful in treating our patients, then the results would speak for themselves. Besides, many people – patients as well as fellow physicians – frown on MDs who advertise. We're very fortunate that word-of-mouth helped build our reputation in Rancho Mirage and in Beverly Hills where our patients became walking advertisements for CSCTC, telling their neighbors and friends about what we do. But word-of-mouth only reaches so far, and there were many patients located far from California who were actively seeking exactly what we had to offer, yet had a tough time finding us. One of those patients is Julia Szabo, a determined New York journalist who spent several years diligently searching the Internet, trying to locate doctors with a treatment protocol exactly like ours.

Even a year after her successful treatment at CSCTC, Julia still shakes her head to think that she could've been treated sooner: "If Dr. Berman and Dr. Lander had advertised, I would've learned about CSCTC faster – and found relief from years of discomfort," she says. "If I'd known about the existence of the Center in 2010, the year it opened, I could have also avoided getting myself into some very unpleasant situations in my quest to be treated with my own stem cells! But they didn't advertise, and the media wasn't doing its job in covering them. So they flew under my radar." Julia wrote about the adventures – and misadventures – of her medical odyssey in a memoir titled *Medicine*

Dog: The Miraculous Cure That Healed My Best Friend and Saved My Life (Lyons Press, 2014). The book chronicles her four-year journey to receive treatment with her own stem cells, which ended positively at our Rancho Mirage office. But before she found us, Julia was obliged first to travel as far away as Panama and Spain in the hope of finding a viable cure for the perirectal fistula which is an aberrant connection between the rectum and the skin that had plagued her since 1999.

By the time she finally did find us, in 2013, Julia had suffered for fourteen years with this lifestyle-hampering condition, which regularly leaked fecal matter into her bloodstream. A fistula is an abnormal passageway, like a tunnel (fistula is Latin for pipe) connecting the inside of the anal canal to the skin around the anus or buttock. The abnormal opening can arise between any two body parts that don't normally connect, but fistulas occur most often in the digestive tract. In 1999, Julia's fistula almost killed her. She was taken to the ER with a high fever and dangerously low blood pressure; she was septic as a result of a perirectal abscess. Sepsis – also known as systemic inflammatory response syndrome, or blood poisoning – is very often a fatal condition, so Julia was fortunate that she was taken to the ER in time.

As her perirectal fistula had leaked infectious matter into her bloodstream, a red, inflamed boil appeared on her right buttock. It was the outer manifestation of what was going on inside: 30 cubic centimeters of pus had collected from the perirectal leakage, and was displacing the tissue of her buttock to create a container for itself. Her body was reacting dramatically to the presence of that pus, which was basically trying to poison her. The ER doctors performed an incision and drainage (I&D for short) to drain the pus; the location of the incision, so near to both the anus and genitalia, made it very difficult to heal. The incision actually never did heal, so Julia was left with not one but two fistulas: the perirectal one, and the one on the inner edge of her right butt-cheek. Julia was also left with many of the symptoms people describe when they have an IBD (inflammatory bowel disease).

People most prone to developing fistulas also suffer from Crohn's disease or ulcerative colitis – collectively termed IBD, for inflammatory bowel disease. Patients with IBD in America number 1.4 million. And yet, surprisingly, too little is written about the day-to-day logistics of struggling with IBD. For patients like Julia, the basic bodily function of defecation is often an excruciating ordeal instead of a relief. It's also quite unpredictable; fecal urgency can strike at any moment, and Murphy's Law seems to dictate that is does so at particularly inconvenient of embarrassing times. Accidentally ingesting one rogue bacterium could result in an unexpected bout of diarrhea, which then results in sepsis, as liquid fecal matter leaks into the bloodstream. There's no way to prevent bacteria from entering the GI tract, so continuous leakage from her rectum into her bloodstream caused Julia to experience the beginnings of sepsis every few months.

A body struggling with sepsis is reacting to bacterial infection that runs rampant through the bloodstream. The system is basically coping with continuous inflammation. That's not a healthy way to live. Julia knew that something had to be done to stop the cycle of infection and re-infection, or she could encounter further health problems as her immune system got tired of battling continuous inflammation. Considering that more than one million Americans live with IBD, one would think that gastrointestinal specialists would be motivated to develop a high-tech treatment method for fistulas. Yet Julia's doctor was recommending a very old-fashioned procedure: a fistulotomy, in which the intestine is tied off with a silk cord (seton) immediately above the abnormal opening that permits infectious matter to breach the bloodstream. This closes off the abnormal opening to prevent further re-infection. The damaged part of the intestine is left to atrophy away, and the patient is left anally incontinent for a period of weeks during healing time.

Julia's main occupational hazard is an insatiable curiosity that fuels her work as a journalist, so she was curious to learn more about fistulotomy by asking questions and doing Internet research. That's how she learned that fistulotomy carries a risk of permanent anal incontinence. It was not uncommon to come across devastated patients who'd undergone the procedure with high hopes, only to emerge with their quality of life seriously compromised. It was a risk Julia refused to take. So she chose to live with her uncomfortable – and potentially fatal – condition. She was hopeful that someday, a more sophisticated fistula treatment method could be found – a twenty-first-century solution to this very old medical problem that had plagued two very famous patients in history: King Louis XIV of France and the author Charles Dickens.

Julia was in luck: The solution she hoped for was being pioneered in Madrid, Spain, where a colorectal surgeon named Damian Garcia-Olmo conducted clinical trials to treat PF patients with their own stem cells. Julia learned of Dr. Garcia-Olmo's groundbreaking work through an unlikely source: her dog. Her main beat as a journalist is pets; she's known as the "Pet Reporter." And in 2008, Julia landed the scoop of her career when she told her readers about Vet-Stem, pioneers in veterinary regenerative medicine. That year, Julia's arthritic dog, a pit bull named Sam, underwent the Vet-Stem procedure and showed immediate and dramatic improvement in his joint strength. Upon realizing that people could not receive stem cell therapy in America at that time, but companion animals could, Julia deduced that, in the United States, veterinary medicine was ahead of human medicine. Her dog could receive treatment with his own stem cells, but she could not. When, a few months later, Time magazine covered Vet-Stem in its July 14, 2008 issue, the headline read: "Stem Cell Therapy for Pets," followed by this: "Sorry, people: A new treatment for ailing joints is only for pooches (and cats and horses)."

Word-of-mouth can work in mysterious ways. If dogs could only talk, Julia would've found us sooner. But since they can't, it took a little longer. By December 2013, Julia's beloved dogs finally led her to our doorstep. The founder of Vet-Stem, Dr. Bob Harman, was one of our earliest patients. He recommended that Julia contact us to make an appointment. And that's how the intrepid Pet Reporter finally achieved her goal – as she puts it, "to be treated like a dog by a doctor as competent as my vet!" As dog lovers ourselves, we have high regard for veterinarians, so we took that as a compliment. After studying Dr. Garcia-Olmo's abstracts on PubMed.com, we decided to put our own stamp on his procedure by adding an IV injection to approach the problem from a local and systemic aspect. The way we performed it, Julia's procedure would be an almost exact replica of the Vet-Stem procedure, which is what her dogs had undergone – and what she wanted for herself from the beginning.

The fact that Julia's surgical wound had never completely healed proved to be a good thing, as it provided an exit pathway for pus to drain away from Julia's body whenever she experienced a relapse, which was often. Every few months or so, she would endure the beginnings of septicemia, complete with extreme exhaustion and abdominal cramping. Our plan was to inject Julia both intravenously and directly into her unhealed surgical wound – with the goal being for the cells to get to work closing the inner fistula first. If the outer fistula were to close up first, infectious matter would have no way to drain away from her body. So, on the day of her treatment, Julia would receive two injections: the first would be delivered intravenously into Julia's bloodstream, and the second would be injected directly into the fistula on her butt-cheek.

The procedure we performed on Julia was not an exact replica of the one pioneered by Dr. Garcia-Olmo in Madrid. He was able to culture his patients' own stem cells to optimize the results, because Europe had no restrictions on the expansion of patients' own cells. However here in America, as we've discussed already, the FDA does not permit what they call "more than minimal manipulation" which is any significant or fundamental alteration of a patient's stem cells. So we performed our own version of the Madrid procedure. Instead of using fibrin glue, as they did in Madrid, we created a custom biologic "glue" out of the platelet-rich plasma in Julia's own blood. It is rich in growth factors and sticky platelets, so we figured it would help her stem cells "stick" to the injection site. In Madrid, the doctors did not administer IV injections of stem cells, but here at CSCTC, we believe that the vascular delivery of cells is, in many cases, the most important part of our process. So, in addition to injecting Julia's cells into her fistula, we also gave her an IV infusion of her stromal vascular fraction which we carefully filter to prevent any clots from forming inside the body.

The success of any stem cell procedure depends on the number of cells extracted from the patient. More fat can mean more stem cells, but unfortunately, Julia didn't have a lot of fat to work with. In fact, when Elliot first met her on the morning of her procedure, he was dismayed to see how slender she was. "I was hoping you'd be fatter!" he said – and he was only half kidding, because of our inability to multiply cells. Happily, Julia's mini-liposuction yielded 42 million viable cells, which we divided in half. The first 21 million cells entered Julia's bloodstream by IV injection. As for the second 21 million, those we injected directly into her exterior fistula.

We weren't sure what to expect from our two-pronged approach, since we had not treated a patient with this problem before. But Julia was confident that, whatever the outcome, she'd be better off for having the procedure done. She has frequently described her experience with stem cells as a "miracle" – in fact, the subtitle of her book is "The Miraculous Cure That Healed My Best Friend and Saved My Life." As scientists, we prefer not to use that type of terminology; we deal in medical practices, not miracles. But we're not surprised that she felt immediately better. Here's how she described that feeling in her book:

> *If I told you that, upon receiving the second injection, I announced that I felt better already, would you believe me? I hardly believed it myself – I'm still a skeptical reporter – but that's precisely what happened. I did feel better already: completely relaxed, as if I'd just had a particularly un-blocking chiropractic adjustment on a sunny beach somewhere. ... The first thing I did upon waking the next morning was – drum roll, please – produce a perfect, pain-free poop.*

We typically tell people to expect healing results anywhere from a few hours to several months after treatment. This is because different cells in the body divide at different rates, so every patient will experience a different result, depending on the condition for which he or she is being treated. Working in Julia's favor was the fact that the area of her body with the most inflammation – the area the stem cells would target for healing – was her gut. It so happens that gut stem cells divide faster than almost any other cell in the body – about every sixteen hours. So, miracles aside, it makes scientific sense that she would feel an improvement almost immediately, and that twelve hours later, she would feel even better still. At long last, Julia's bowels were complying with her for the first time in almost fifteen years. That first post-treatment bowel movement was so epic for Julia that she took a photograph of it with her iPhone and emailed the picture to us! Certainly one of our most unusual post op photos we've seen in our careers. To this day, Julia has enjoyed normal bowel function.

In the end, with all due respect to Julia and other patients who tell us to advertise, we weren't wrong: Usually it was word-of-mouth that would lead our patients to us. We just never imagined that word could spread so efficiently from the non-speaking mouth of a loyal dog! The moral? Always go with your gut.

Chapter 10

CONFRONTING OUR CRITICS

At the California Stem Cell Treatment Center®, we're all admirers of the controversial author and philosopher Ayn Rand. In Rand's bestselling 1957 novel *Atlas Shrugged*, the central protagonists are characters who all share a strong sense of self-esteem, self-worth, and the kind of selfishness that is widely misunderstood. Their names are Francisco, Ragnar, and Hank. (Of course, the elusive John Galt is the story's ultimate hero, but for most of the novel we only hear about him, not from him: "*Who is John Galt?*" is the very first line of the book and an oft-repeated refrain throughout.) These people are self-starters, and their successes – resulting from their own industry and initiative – provide them with their own rewards, regardless of what others may think.

Rand's characters are so good at what they do, that they become the targets of complicated ploys to take them down, or force them to stand on equal footing with far less enterprising, less hard-working individuals. In *Atlas Shrugged*, for instance, Congress manipulates the laws so as to require entrepreneurs – notably Hank, inventor of a versatile alloy called Rearden Metal – to give away the very innovations they developed because, well, it's "only fair" to spread the wealth – isn't it? Today, we are reminded of the nefarious nature of income inequality. If we're all created equally, then why don't we all share the same income levels – isn't that "only fair"? And nobody really invented anything on their own, the "government" provided the support and infra-structure, so we should all share in these "personal" accomplishments – right?

So, what are we getting at? Any time someone – whether in an Ayn Rand novel or in "real" life – puts forward an effort that flies in the face of conformity, the critics will object. And worse, if the non-conformist is successful, others will claim that his or her success belongs, not to the individualist, but to the majority. Rand herself experienced this, and although she died in 1982, she and her work continue to draw heated criticism. We can relate: From the start of our venture into the deployment of adipose derived stromal vascular fraction (SVF), we have been treated to an uninterrupted stream of criticism. After all, what right do we have to use these adipose cells to investigate therapeutic applications, and to charge for our services before the protocol has been proven (by whom?) to be successful?

Early criticisms came from our own colleagues. They generally complained that we didn't know if SVF deployment was safe or any better than a placebo. While we cared that treatments were effective, we focused our initial study on safety by looking at adverse events. If it weren't safe, why would we venture into this area? Of course, a plethora of empirical and anecdotal data existed suggesting safety would not be an issue. Nonetheless, stories of calamities related to "stem cell" deployments would arise from time to time, make it into the press or the online chat sites and get disseminated throughout the medical community and general public. People could be easily scared. Nonetheless, our first study focused on any adverse events. While there were the occasional complaints about the liposuction (mainly that there was some pain at the site after surgery), there were no significant adverse events (complications) directly related to the administration of SVF. Of course, we expected this. These cells came from the same person, were just released in larger numbers, procured in a completely sterile manner, filtered through a 100 micron filter, and if administered intravenously they passed through an intravenous filter for blood (170 micron). Thus, there was no chance of infection or clotting from an embolus.

The second predominant line of criticism came from doctors who admonished us for not performing evidence-based studies with placebos. "You don't know if this is any better than a placebo," they exclaimed in fairly standard response. Initially, we weren't too interested in doing controlled studies; we just wanted to see if SVF really worked in any consistent manner. We wanted to see if some of the claims and testimonials made throughout scattered clinics around the world had any merit while validating the safety of the procedure. If all went well, then we would do more formal studies as we progressed forward. If it didn't work, then case closed, and we'd venture no further.

As you may recall, we started by looking at orthopedic cases. Most of our patients that suffered from joint degeneration had already had multiple treatments – e.g. NSAID (non-steroidal anti-inflammatory) pain medicines, steroid injections, hyaluronic acid injections, and even arthroplasty – yet they didn't get better. Of course, if they didn't get better from treatments they expected to help them, they obviously didn't get better from any placebo effect that could have possibly occurred from a proposed therapy. However, early on we found that these same patients responded positively to SVF. It would be highly unlikely that SVF has any better of a placebo effect than any other received therapy. Thus, it would be illogical to suggest that improvement following SVF could be due to a placebo. Eventually, we'll have to have some controlled studies to support these findings. In the meantime, patients are seeking relief from years of pain – and we believe it's our empiric evidence that helps us focus our efforts on therapy and optimization of therapy.

As we started to grow the Cell Surgical Network®, we started to garner more attention. Although many colleagues questioned why we hadn't yet published any papers in scientific journals, other colleagues that knew us or heard us speak became interested in joining up with our team. We slowly and organically started forming a network of doctors dedicated to investigational deployments of SVF. Unfortunately, our colleagues, while attending various stem cell conferences, have reported that some of the speakers had lumped us in with other organizations doing stem cell work and then proceeded to vilify us. A well-known bioethicist declared that we were "unethical" and practicing without FDA approval. We went ahead and established a professional dialogue with this bioethicist, and tried to explain our position both as surgeons and with respect to the FDA regulations that govern "Human, Cells, Tissues, and Tissue and Cell Based Products (HCT/Ps)."

We stand by the premise of our practice: The protocol of the Cell Surgical Network® – investigational deployments of SVF for therapeutic purposes – is not FDA-approved, but it is FDA-compliant, and hence, entirely ethical.

While this dialogue occurred in a very polite email environment, we could never get the abovementioned bioethicist to understand or agree with our position. And, it turns out, without having mentioned it, this bioethicist had actually reported us to the FDA as an organization that needed to be looked into and potentially shut down. Ironically, he had sent this letter in January 2013, at least 10 months prior to our conversation, yet never mentioned it to us during our conversations. We tried to explain that we perform a surgical procedure and the FDA has no jurisdiction over the practice of surgery. The FDA has jurisdiction over drugs and devices. Once a device or drug has been approved for any claim, a surgeon may use said drug or device in any manner they see fit. Momentarily, we will go into detail about the FDA issue, so that it's well understood – even though there will doubtless be criticism even of this explanation.

After doing an interview with a noted PhD stem cell blogger, we were summarily dismissed for our "violation" of FDA regulations and accused of taking advantage of our patients for monetary gain. Simply, we were noted to be greedy doctors preying upon desperate patients.

The FDA continues to effectively and ethically do exactly what Congress mandated them to do, which is protect society from the transmission of disease by regulating our food and medicine supply. The vocal PhD critics, on the other hand, are using their prestigious credentials and titles ("Bioethicist," "Medical Ethicist") to appoint themselves watchdogs of the stem cell industry. This is, we believe, the opposite of ethical. For decades, physician practices, research, and overall behavior have been closely regulated and controlled by medical boards, peer review, insurance companies, local laws, malpractice attorneys, patient groups, hospitals, and various other regulators. It is only very recently that grant-receiving biologists have suddenly stepped up to "protect" patients from physicians. We would suggest to these "ethicists" that they are neither qualified nor entitled to regulate physicians. They should engage primarily in peer review and focus on irreproducible results from various "prestigious" labs, or on the 261 stem cell lines in the NIH that have not been cleared for sterility (E.C. Jonlin, "Differing standards for the NIH Stem Cell Registry and FDA approval render most federally funded hESC lines unsuitable for clinical use," *Cell Stem Cell*, 14:139-40, 2014), but have been used in research for commercialization for more than twelve years. Such endeavors are the most appropriate for these "ethicists" if they truly want to be involved in "protecting" patients.

One thing about CSCTC® and CSN®, we don't back down and we're not afraid to take on the negative press. Why? Understanding the FDA rules and regulations, and how they have been manipulated by self-interested individuals and groups, is only part of the reason why we comfortably confront our critics. The main reason we can comfortably stand up for our position is our commitment to carrying out our duties as physicians. Our responsibility is a substantial one: to come to the aid of our patients whenever possible. It is, or should be, a fundamental responsibility of all practicing physicians. If you can help them, then you should provide the effort.

So, how is it that the FDA regulations have been cited to suggest that we are out of bounds in providing investigational deployment of SVF? For this we need a little history lesson, as well as an understanding of FDA responsibilities. First, to be clear, the FDA, with respect to medicine, has always been responsible for two things: drugs and devices. In order for a drug or device to be approved, it must go through FDA-approved tests that ultimately show a reasonable degree of safety and efficacy (effectiveness). Indeed, there are many very useful drugs that can help a large number of patients, yet may actually kill a small (and "acceptable") number of patients, who may experience an allergic response or sustain some other serious harm as a result of taking the drug. Further, drugs that help most people might not actually be effective for a select group of patients.

Nonetheless, if the drugs' claims are reasonable, they can be FDA approved. Nearly every medication and device carries certain known risks, even though FDA-approved disclosures about these risks must be made. Once a drug or device has been approved for any claim, medical doctors – surgeons as well as physicians – can use those products in any capacity they see fit. *Therefore, there are NO "FDA-approved" surgical procedures.* And the FDA does not limit doctors as to how we may use an approved drug or device. The only limit on drugs and devices relates to how a company may fairly advertise their product to physicians and to the public.

For example, the uber-popular drug Botox has long been used to wipe out a large variety of facial wrinkles. The product was originally developed and approved for use in blepharospasm (uncontrolled eyelid twitching). Eventually, while Botox was used for several different facial wrinkles, the company eventually got FDA clearance for the correction or softening of the glabellar wrinkle (the frown lines between your eyes). Of course, the drug is used for multiple wrinkles other than the frown wrinkle, yet no one voices concern that it's not approved for these other wrinkles. The Federal Trade Commission and Federal Communications Commission weren't pleased with the Botox Cosmetic advertisements that seemed to promote Botox without specifying its actual claims, and suggested it could simply support any kind of cosmetic enhancement. The ads were eventually pulled, but still medical doctors are free to use Botox any way they see fit.

This actually makes a lot of sense. It would be overwhelming for a drug or device manufacturer to satisfy every possible claim that could arise from any of its products. Aspirin, for example, may have been approved as a headache remedy, but as a blood thinner, it has become an important medication for heart and stroke patients, and patients at potential risk from clotting. Some studies suggest there are other benefits beyond these, but what aspirin manufacturer wants to pursue every claim? Scientists and doctors may see empirical evidence of the value of aspirin, and may thus set up a variety of studies to support or reject such hypothesis, but the companies need not set up more studies to make more claims. If there's a significant financial advantage, then they might pursue new claims; otherwise they'll be content to let the medical community drive sales of their product.

In 2001, the U.S. Congress passed a law that mandated the FDA to set up regulations for the purpose of preventing disease transmission in the exchange of body parts. In particular, there existed concern over organ donations, whereby a number of recipients had succumbed to HIV, hepatitis, and other serious infections after successful transplantation of donated organs. Congress wanted someone to police or regulate such tissue transfers, to minimize or eliminate risks of disease transmission. 21 Code of Federal Regulations part 1271 emerged in 2005, providing a set of guidelines for which the FDA could claim jurisdiction over human body parts. It may seem strange that in America, a government body could establish any regulations as to how its citizens may use their own body parts; however, Congress asked the FDA to do just that. If you read the first page of this regulation, you actually learn that the purpose of this rule is to "prevent the transmission of communicable disease." In order to do this, the FDA must define when they have jurisdiction over your tissues – i.e. they must meet the definition of a drug or device.

The FDA came up with a list of exemptions that would allow doctors to circumvent the need for formal FDA approval through filing an Investigational New Drug application. If all of the following criteria were met, then a doctor or medical organization would be free to treat a patient with an HCT/P (Human Cells, Tissues, and Cellular and Tissue-Based Products). These exemptions include: 1) the parts must be autologous (from the same person); 2) for homologous use (used as the same tissue); 3) done during the same surgical setting; 4) minimally manipulated; 5) not labeled (e.g. can't make claims, provide testimonials, or advertised promotions), and 6) can't be used for systemic effects unless a) autologous, b) from a primary relative, or c) used for reproductive purposes.

Now, what our critics fail to understand is that if there is any risk of disease transmission, then the FDA must invoke its jurisdiction, and it must support its position by showing that the process in question comes under its jurisdiction. To date, the FDA has shut down several clinics and laboratories. In all cases, they visited the site and found violations of GMP (Good Manufacturing Practices): manufacturing that could jeopardize sterility. As such, these organizations were told to "clean up" to FDA standards and close their doors until they were in compliance. One well-known group from Colorado that was using a laboratory for their technology decided to sue the FDA because they believed that the FDA had no jurisdiction over the practice of medicine. However, the FDA, by virtue of the Congressional law, was given the responsibility to prevent disease transmission, and when a laboratory gets involved, the FDA exerts its jurisdiction over the production process.

The lawsuit against the FDA failed in part because the FDA simply argued that it had jurisdiction over these organizations that violated GMP procedures. To cite its jurisdiction, it showed a list of its regulations. The company "cultured stem cells in their lab" and because this was arguably "more than minimal manipulation" – plus, the same company provided testimonials and made claims, thereby "labeling" its product – then the FDA had jurisdiction. The courts upheld the FDA position. The courts agreed that this particular medical group could harvest cells from patients and provide them back to the same patients – but it ventured outside a "point of care" delivery, the laboratory expansion (culturing to grow more cells) came under the FDA jurisdiction, and thus had to prove there was no risk of disease transmission.

For a variety of reasons that we can imagine, but in this context will not speculate upon, the same organization in conflict with the FDA had colleagues send correspondence to the FDA asking if approval could be granted for using "collagenase to process autologous lipo-aspirate (the fat from liposuction) to produce stem cells." In such circumstances, the FDA must review and respond to these requests. They evaluate these notes in a committee referred to as a Tissue Reference Group (TRG). They are not legal documents, but do represent the opinion of the FDA. We can tell you that if we worked at the FDA we would not approve any such note, and we use collagenase to process our cells. Why? Such open-ended letters are rather deceptive. While they may sound fairly clear, too much is missing in order to provide an affirmative response. If the FDA doesn't know how the cells are processed, the source of the collagenase, or other significant details, then any letter of affirmation would be tantamount to "FDA approval." If a calamity later occurred, then these physicians could claim that they had been vetted and essentially approved by the FDA.

One such TRG letter that cast false aspersions on the use of collagenase was written by a physician related to the abovementioned Colorado group, which focuses exclusively on the use of bone marrow as a source of stem cells. Using bone marrow cells does not include the use of collagenase, which is only used to procure fat-derived stem cells and subsequently, that TRG letter – which was well-circulated by the marketing department of the Colorado organization – undermined the efforts of those using fat, creating an unfair marketing advantage. The abuse of the regulatory process for economic benefit is prevalent in many new scientific fields and the stem cell world is no different. Most commonly used collagenases are "laboratory grade" and manufactured as bovine (cow) byproducts. Bovine products aren't screened or prepared to prevent transmissible spongiform encephalopathies (TSEs), more commonly known as the cause of "mad cow disease." As such, there's no way the FDA, without knowing exact details about the collagenase, could safely give permission for such manipulation. The type of collagenase that we use is prepared by Roche Laboratories from a specially cultured bacterium by GMP standards and carries no risk of disease transmission.

Clearly, in such a case as described, the FDA has too much to risk and virtually nothing to gain. It's comprised of humans who don't want to be caught up in such potential legal battles. However, rather than understanding that these FDA "disapprovals" are meant to protect the public from disease transmission, the "word" throughout the medical and scientific community has been adulterated to suggest that the FDA can stop anyone that deviates from any of the above noted "exemptions." Of course, if this were the case, any physician using cells or tissues that are "more than minimally manipulated" or not used as a "homologous" part could be sanctioned by the FDA. However, in surgery, we frequently use tissues that are more than minimally manipulated, and we use them in non-homologous areas. For example, a burn might be covered by a skin graft that has been run through a device that cuts into it so severely that it can be stretched to cover a larger surface area. Such "meshed" grafts are extremely manipulated, but the FDA would never interfere in their use.

Collagenase, the drug in the middle of this controversy, only affects the collagen tissue that binds the cells together. It doesn't even enter a phospholipid cell membrane. As such, there's no manipulation of the cells, just the non-cellular collagen. Yet our critics will suggest we are more than minimally manipulating the tissue, because the FDA suggested such in their TRG response. We firmly believe that the FDA takes this position because it can't determine how the collagenase was manufactured, nor how it's being used. Further, collagenase is already available as an FDA-approved drug for use in a couple of well-known medical conditions. The drug can simply be injected directly into the body without any issue at all, as it's already FDA approved. When we use it, we completely wash it out from our final product, yet there are those concerned that some collagenase could get into the body and be harmful. Are they serious? Our studies with Roche show no significantly measurable collagenase left in the SVF; our critics countered that some residual collagenase could be getting into the body – yet you're already allowed to inject massive doses of collagenase directly into one's body for known conditions. Talk about silly arguments. Recall that, as surgeons, we are allowed to use any approved drug or device any way we deem necessary, regardless of the exact claims approved. Recent FDA draft guidance documents cite collagenase and any other method of fat digestion as "more than minimally manipulated." This proves that collagenase was never the issue. It was always about the FDA having jurisdiction over any type of fat digestion IF there was a risk of transmissible disease.

Our critics also like to point out that we are not using the SVF cells for homologous purposes. See the "History of SVF" section at the end of this book to see evidence that SVF can form any kind of tissue, defying the strict definition of "homologous." Of course, if the cells help grow new cartilage or restore vascular or nerve function it seems pretty obvious that they are being used to do what they're supposed to do – namely, differentiate into the needed cells or tissues. Nonetheless, as surgeons, we routinely use cells or tissues for non-homologous purposes. We'll give you some simple examples. Start with a very popular procedure: coronary artery bypass grafting. This procedure is frequently performed using veins to replace arteries. That's non-homologous. We've also been performing fat transfer procedures since the 1980s. While we mostly use fat to help repair fat loss from aging in the face, it has also been used for non-homologous purposes, such as filling in defects from muscle tissue losses or filling in breast defects after resection or radiation damage to breast tissue. A bladder removed because of cancer or some other damage can be reconstructed with a section of ileum (small intestine). These are all non-homologous surgical procedures, over which the FDA has no jurisdiction.

We produce SVF in a completely closed, sterile, "surgical" environment, using approved drugs and devices without any risk of disease transmission – yet our critics remain adamant that we are somehow in violation of 21 CFR part 1271, and the FDA should shut us down. In fact, some of these critics have even written to the FDA as far back as January 2013, yet the FDA has not taken any action against us. Still, that doesn't stop our critics, who have also called upon other scientists and doctors to write more letters to the FDA complaining about their "perceived violations on our part."

Ironically, we've actually been in close contact with the FDA, as we are pursuing FDA approval for our "device system" for producing SVF. We don't have a singular device but rather a surgical system. As such, we planned some straightforward investigations to test the safety and efficacy (effectiveness) of our system. Through conversations and our pre-IDE meetings with the FDA, they provided us guidance on how to best achieve our approval for the TimeMachine® (the SVF devices we trademarked from Korea). We are not flying under FDA radar, and we run absolutely no risk of disease transmission from our handling procedures. Indeed, we've sent multiple tissue samples of SVF out for evaluation, and have never had a positive response (i.e. any contamination with bacteria). Thus, we have no real issues with the FDA in spite of the critics.

It's actually sad to see how so many scientists and physicians have been manipulated by special interest groups that have used the FDA to falsely support their position, keep out competition, and prevent doctors like us from simply caring for our patients. Indeed, as physicians, we appreciate that the Hippocratic oath (and the AMA code of ethics) are pretty clear about a doctor's responsibility to help his/her patients if at all possible. Further, while we have plenty of knowledge to support the use of SVF, all of our patients and affiliates recognize that, during this early stage of cell deployment, we are still "investigating" the results. We are amassing a lot of empirical data that will help us improve delivery of cell therapy to a variety of conditions and learn about SVF and its ability to correct (or not correct) a variety of inflammatory and degenerative conditions.

Another criticism we frequently get is that we are charging our patients while doing investigative work. That's very true, except for the patients to whom we give big discounts or treat for free. The FDA actually allows doctors to charge (not gouge) reasonable fees for investigative work. During the silicone gel investigation (1992-2007), the breast implant manufacturers were still making on the order of $300 million USD each year. Also, citizens putting up their own money privately fund our work. In California, CIRM (California Institute for Regenerative Medicine) has spent nearly $2 billion USD funding a variety of research programs with public money. Imagine, the taxpayer has supported the building of large offices and laboratories on some campuses, where their endowments are in excess of $16 billion USD. How ethical is that? The PhDs are getting paid no matter whether they help someone or not. We would have stopped a long time ago if our work was fruitless or in any way harmful. While not everyone gets better from SVF deployment, so many do improve that we find ourselves in the midst of the most rewarding time of our careers: We're doing precisely what we dreamed of doing when, back in college, we answered the calling to become medical doctors. We doubt we could ever return to the sidelines now, after seeing how we've helped so many people, using their own restorative cells to restore function and eliminate pain.

Disruptive isn't always a negative term – especially when it's used to describe a phenomenon that shakes up an existing order that's become outdated, or has reached the limits of its potential to help people. Our disruptive technology may very well lead to the use of routine autologous SVF in every medical center in the world, as an adjunct to current standard medical therapies. This is all occurring years, even decades, before stem cell therapies provided by the pharmaceutical industry – "Big Pharma" – make their appearance in our medical practices. It's no wonder that our work has stirred so much anxiety among many so-called "experts in the field." When we first began to field particularly vitriolic opposition to our investigative work with SVF, we wondered, "What are they so afraid of?" The answer to that question should trouble some of our prominent "bio-ethicist" critics much more than questions such as "Is it ethical to charge patients?"

So, while our critics continue to predict our demise and call for our dismissal, we "fight on," honestly surprised that anyone would be upset with us for actually trying to help patients. We don't dismiss the great work being contributed by our Ph.D. colleagues, and we imagine that, at some point, someone will hand us these "magic cells" in a bottle and we'll be able to simply use them and forgo our procedure. We believe there will likely exist the desire to use your own DNA and freeze and store (cryo-preserve) your own cells for later use – both to restore damaged tissues and regenerate naturally degrading tissues. This will not only restore function and eliminate pain, but will eventually be a source for prolonging life well into the 100's.

In recent months, we have answered several invitations to speak at medical meetings or help set up autologous cell therapy practices in the USA and abroad. We've been working with regulatory authorities in China, the European Union, and Australia to help create policies regarding the use of autologous cell therapies. Critics often wonder why we haven't published our treatment results in peer-reviewed medical journals, and cite this as "proof" of our "lack of ethics"; we've prepared a manuscript for review that encompasses the safety and efficacy experience with our first thousand patients. But as we've said before, we don't believe it would be ethical to stop treating patients until after the article is published; we want to help patients as soon as possible.

Without courting the attention of the mainstream media, we did not court the fourth estate's attention, but now reporters from television, newspaper, and magazine outlets are contacting us, wanting to know more. Amongst them was CBS News, "The Doctors" show, and Associated Press. The June 2015 issue of *Popular Science* magazine had an excellent article on California Stem Cell Treatment Center and the Network. Our affiliate in Ohio, cosmetic surgeon Dr. Mark Foglietti, was featured on his local news station for treating two high-profile patients. In February 2014, Fox8 Cleveland did an inspiring profile on popular radio personality Kym Sellers of Cleveland's Radio One, WZAK, 93.1. Kym has advanced Multiple Sclerosis, and heads the Kym Sellers Foundation, whose motto is "Live Long, Fight Strong, 'Til MS is Gone." Early in 2014, she decided to undergo investigational stem cell therapy with Dr. Foglietti. In April 2014, the Fox8 did a follow-up report in which Kym's doctors described their famous patient's progress as a "remarkable response," with improvements to her breathing and range of motion.

Kym's story, in turn, inspired another local hero to consult Dr. Foglietti: former Cleveland Browns player Joe Jurevicius. At 39, the retired wide receiver's knees were going to require total replacement, but he chose autologous stem cell therapy instead. We were particularly impressed when the Fox8 reporter, Suzanne Stratford, referenced a pop-culture phenomenon to help viewers understand how stem cells work: she described them as "microscopic Transformers." That's a very helpful and impactful way to understand ASCs.

Media coverage of the Cell Surgical Network® isn't always positive, however. Dr. Steven Gitt was interviewed for television by Nancy Snyderman, NBC's Chief Medical Editor. In her interview, Ms. Snyderman asked Dr. Gitt – a well-known plastic surgeon with superlative credentials, practicing with our network in Arizona – what "right" he had to be doing this kind of work, since investigational stem cell work should be done in a university. Since then, her reporter's judgment came into question when, in a scene that could've been scripted by Ayn Rand, Ms. Snyderman violated her own Ebola virus quarantine to sneak out for a meal with her camera crew. Ms. Snyderman has since resigned and it is notable that her interview of Dr. Gitt originally aired on the (who else but?) Brian Williams segment of NBC news.

We never know what direction a media story might take, or whether it will be positive or critical. But what we do know is that we had come to the end of the year, and our practice and network was still standing – yet its demise had been predicted for this year, 2014, by our "stem cell blogger" in his January "forecasts" for the New Year. In *Atlas Shrugged*, the plot lines all intersect with a fictitious, New York-based railway enterprise called Taggart Transcontinental. We think of the Cell Surgical Network® as a bullet train to the future of medicine, transporting patients to an improved quality of life. CSN has grown to more than 85 affiliate physician groups in the United States and abroad, and it's still growing. The train has left the station.

ADDENDUM –
THE NEWSPAPER CRITICS

On September 9, 2013, *The New York Times* – the "newspaper of record" and a tremendously powerful influencer of public opinion – published an article by Laura Beil entitled "Stem Cell Treatments Overtake Science." We found the article to be heavily biased against the use of adult stem cells from fat. Although our practice was not mentioned, we promptly wrote a letter to the editor. Our letter was never published, and to date the *Times* has not approached us for input into an article about adult stem cell therapy.

What follows below is our response to the *Times* – and what follows after that? The stories of how and why we started our practice, and the patients whose successes with stem cell therapy inspire us every day.

"Stem Cell Treatments Overtake Science"
by LAURA BEIL
Published in *The New York Times* September 9, 2013

(Unpublished) Response by Mark Berman, MD and Elliot Lander, MD
California Stem Cell Treatment Center

Rancho Mirage, CA

September 12, 2013

To the Editor:

It's clear from Ms. Beil's article that there is confusion between junk science and junk medicine. We're always a bit concerned when we read about PhD's concerned about real science and bioethics. Doctors have a responsibility to take care of their patients. Definitely, the promotion of "snake oil" products and pure hucksterism should be frowned upon. However, there is NO DOUBT that doctors can isolate cells from fat and other body tissues that are incredibly rich in regenerative cells (many of which are adult stem cells). Also, there is little doubt that these cells can provide an incredible resource to mend inflammatory or degenerative conditions. Such work has been demonstrated time and again with evidenced-based (i.e. scientific) studies in Europe and even in the United States, though predominantly in the veterinary industry. While unscrupulous practitioners may "prey upon the public," let us remind you that there is no industry as thoroughly regulated as medicine – with oversight at multiple levels, not the least of which is through the legal system.

The Cell Surgical Network® (www.stemcellrevolution.com) supports a number of affiliates throughout the United States and abroad that provide a simple closed surgical technique to provide deployment of adult regenerative cells from a mini-liposuction procedure under an IRB approved protocol. We are registered with Clinical Trials.gov through the National Institutes of Health (NIH). We house a huge online database and will likely publish findings of our initial safety studies within the next six months (trials of any kind take time). Transparency remains the foundation on which we base our efforts. Patients know from the start that they may not obtain positive results. Not infrequently, this is simply due to a poor harvest of regenerative cells and patients are offered repeat treatments at little or no cost under a variety of conditions.

We contend that if you read the AMA code of ethics, we meet every criterion for an ethical practice. Further, our primary team (the California Stem Cell Treatment Center) and all of our affiliates have been built upon a multidisciplinary team approach. Our Board Certified doctors cover multiple specialties including plastic surgery, orthopedic surgery, cardiology, urology, interventional radiology, neurosurgery, spine specialists, ophthalmologists, and others. All are highly respected and considered thought leaders in their respective fields. This is hardly an organization built on the backs of some nefarious underground community that wants to remain anonymous.

While we appreciate the need for evidence-based studies, please understand that empirical medicine is NOT USELESS. Our scientists have been housed in glorious laboratories for years now with little clinical data to show for their efforts. We know that we can help people now with their own cells, amazingly richly found in adipose tissue. Why not do it? It might not be safe, we're told. So, we're doing a study that studies safety as the primary objective. Barely three years and one thousand patients into the study, there are no signs of significant adverse events short of occasional complaints about soreness around the liposuction site (which is actually an expected sequelae).

Our secondary objective is to look at clinical outcomes and see if we can identify trends. Of course, we've seen incredible results in a vast number of patients. Yet, the pundits will retort that because patients may pay for treatment (and there are many that get their treatment for free) there may be a significant placebo effect and our results are valueless. Most of our patients, particularly with orthopedic conditions, have already had a multitude of treatments before they come to us for cell deployment. If someone paid money for an accepted treatment and didn't get better, clearly the treatment wasn't effective. Of course, every treatment, paid for or not, has a potential placebo effect. So, if after four or five failed treatments the patient actually gets better from cell deployment, why would the placebo effect be any greater from cell deployment than any previous treatment? It's not logical to assume that any treatment has a greater placebo effect. Yet we see this assumption made frequently.

We also would argue that as we make headway with empirical successes, it will be easier for scientists to go back to the laboratory to understand why and how we can improve on the process. We have a Hippocratic duty to help our patients now simply because we can. "I will prescribe regimens for the good of my patients according to my ability and my judgment." We don't need to wait until someone builds a "better mouse-trap" when we have a "mouse-trap" that already works. When they build a better one, we'll all gladly switch to it.

Unfortunately, the public is being bamboozled by big business, big pharma, big universities, and any organization that has a lot at stake in this multi-billion dollar industry of stem cells. Their regard for our patients is rather disingenuous when they tell the public they're worried about bad results killing the industry. That's hardly a risk. The cream always rises to the top, as we've seen time and again with medical procedures and good medical discoveries. If it really works, doctors and patients eventually catch on. If it doesn't, it becomes a footnote in history. The truly unscrupulous characters ultimately get weeded out.

EPILOGUE

What does the future hold?

At this point we want to roll out our big crystal ball that predicts the future of stem cell therapies. We think that regenerative medicine will advance greatly but slowly over the next ten years and that cell therapy will continue to evolve into two main arenas. One will be the long term research and monetization of patents in parallel with the development of therapies that can be mass produced in corporate laboratories to create a "stem cells in a bottle" type of product. The other arena will contain cell based therapies using autologous cells isolated from the human body as the ultimate production laboratory in a point of care system of cell therapy. This second system has tremendous potential to influence the way medical care is delivered in the US and around the entire world obviating the need for multimillion dollar laboratories, patents, and delivery of care through big Pharma-based models. This is why we are calling this the Stem Cell Revolution® and it is a disruptive technology.

Our hope and vision is that cell therapy will be available to clinicians and every medical clinic based on simple, safe, sterile procedures and tissue transfer principles that we use every day in surgery. We hope and believe that these therapies will be affordable and reliable. Our early research has shown excellent safety but we find that many patients (especially those with neurodegenerative and auto-immune conditions) need repeat treatments requiring multiple liposuctions adding to the expense and hassle of autologous treatments. However, we have been actively working from a scientific and regulatory perspective on finding methods of cryogenically freezing stromal vascular fraction so that multiple deployments can be provided economically and conveniently. Further, we believe that all adults should consider donating a small amount of their fat to a bio-bank that could preserve it for future needs – i.e. as bio-insurance. Currently, technology exists it freeze SVF and immortalize one's cells. Even more exciting, we can expand and grow them; effectively creating a nearly unlimited supply of a person's own healing stem cells that may be critical should one develop cancer, an illness, or suffer from trauma. Additionally, these expanded cells may be instrumental in prolonging vital longevity. To realize this potential, we have created "Cells On Ice"™, working in conjunction with American CryoStem. Just as parents have been saving umbilical tissue for their children's "bio-insurance", we think many adults would like to put their own "cells on ice" in the same way. Indeed, fat may have even greater potential than umbilical tissue.

The idea of using one's cells to fight cancer might not seem too likely. However, stem cells have the distinct advantage of homing in on cancer tissues in an attempt to repair the damage caused by malignant growth. This feature may be exploited to carry cancer killing chemotherapy and biologic agents directly to the tumor microenvironment, essentially acting as a "Trojan horse" to improve the delivery of such agents. We strongly believe that having a deposit of your own cells available to you on a moment's notice should you have an accident, heart attack, stroke or sudden illness would provide you with a type of biologic health insurance superior in quality and at a fraction of the price to traditional health insurance.

All of the technology needed to cryogenically freeze and replicate your cells and then safely deliver them back to you already exists. See www. cellsonice.com

We predict that your own stem cells – whether fresh or frozen or ultimately expanded – will be routinely used for a variety of conditions not currently considered. For example, we believe that they could be used post-operatively for nearly every orthopedic operation, as they should help you mend much better and much quicker from injury or surgery. They will likely become a source of first intervention in heart attack, stroke and head trauma. Not only will they be used routinely to help athletes mend better and quicker, but may even be considered to help them maximize their potential. And lastly, for age mitigation strategies, one can continuously re-deploy expanded autologous cells to simply replace normally dying cells thus continually replenishing and restoring your vital organs and tissues. These cells could essentially be your ticket to a vital and functional increase in life-span. A crystal ball isn't necessary to see how these cells can be incredibly useful, but it may be necessary to see what kind of cells – your own or those processed in a laboratory – are going to be most functional. We believe that even if allogeneic cells (someone else's) become available and well accepted, there will always be a benefit (unless you have a genetic defect) to receiving your own DNA.

It's exciting to know that in many respects the future is here. There will be continued new discoveries and therefore the demand will likely increase with time.

END NOTE

Has a doctor ever told you "there's nothing we can do"? We sincerely hope you won't accept that as the final answer, because as doctors, we believe that there's always something you can do. Our physician colleagues in the Cell Surgical Network are now treating a wide range of conditions, many of which previously had "no treatment options" – below is a list, in alphabetical order. To locate the doctor nearest you, visit www.cellsurgicalnetwork.com

ALS
Alzheimer's
Alopecia Areata
Arrhythmia
Arthritis and degenerative Orthopedic conditions
Asthma
Autism
Autoimmune Hepatitis Diabetes Mellitus
Autoimmune Neuropathy
Cerebral Palsy
CIDP (Chronic Inflammatory Demyelinating Polyneuropathy)
Congestive Heart Failure
COPD/Emphysema
Critical Limb Ischemia
Crohn's Disease
Dermatomyositis
Dry eyes
Erectile Dysfunction
Fibromyalgia

Glaucoma
Hashimoto's Thyroiditis
Interstitial Cystitis
Lichen Sclerosus
Lung Disease
Lupus
Lymphedema
Macular Degeneration
Male Incontinence
Ménière's
Multiple Sclerosis
Muscular Dystrophy
Myasthenia Gravis
Myocardial Infarction
Optic Neuritis
Parkinson's
Peyronies
Polychondritis
Post Radical Prostatectomy
Rectal Fistula
Renal Failure
Retinopathy
Rheumatoid Arthritis
Scleroderma
Severe Peripheral Arterial Disease
Spasmodic Dysphonia
Stroke
Traumatic Brain Injury and Concussion

ACKNOWLEDGMENTS

This entire book represents an acknowledgment. Everyone mentioned in the book is the backbone for the story and we thank them all for their contributions. However, a few people not mentioned need to be and maybe a few of those mentioned should be further acknowledged.

The process of writing a book is laborious at best. We'd like to start by thanking Julia Szabo who co-wrote, organized, co-edited and conducted all of the interviews so that we could give our voice yet present our patients in an impartial manner without coaching them. Julia has written her own best-seller, *Medicine Dog: The Miraculous Cure That Healed My Best Friend and Saved My Life*. Perhaps too, we should thank her dog who ultimately brought her to us via Bob Harman, president of Vet-Stem. Vet-Stem has treated over 10,000 animals from poodles to thoroughbred horses using adipose derived cells. We established a wonderful relationship with Bob Harman whose efforts helped us advance our technique to its current status – completely closed sterile surgical procedure with filtered cells.

The labor of writing this book reflects the somewhat divine intervention afforded to us through the special people we have met, worked with and ultimately became part of the CSCTC and CSN team. There would have been no book and no entry into SVF without the genius of Dr. Hee Young Lee. As mentioned in the book, Dr. Lee is medicine's version of Tony Stark from the Ironman movie. His most clever inventions are the foundation for our venture into therapeutic stem cell deployment. However, we would never have known of Dr. Lee had it not been for the tireless work of Peter Jung. Additionally, Steven Hwang, along with the rest of the Medikhan team has been invaluable with their efforts in helping us see this project into fruition.

We have been honored to have Jackie See MD, highly respected interventional cardiologist and stem cell pioneer, join our clinical research project when we first started out. He gave freely of his abundant knowledge and helped us shape our vision of regenerative medicine while always reminding us of the physician's role to remain the ultimate patient advocate.

We'd like to acknowledge the special contributions from our office staff. On the administrative side - Judi Meglio, Marlina Manchego, Annette Pinuelas, Chris Lindholm, Lauren Geddie, Nikki Mitchell and Raziq Noorali. In the surgical suite, Aylin Soleymanian, Jessica Valdez, Brittany Whitley, Shawntae Dowell, and Elideili Villicana have been instrumental in forwarding our techniques. Aylin, in particular, was there when we started and helped devise a lot of the modifications we added to Dr. Lee's original system.

Finally, we'd like to thank those initial patients – the true pioneers that trusted us to try their own SVF to improve their conditions. In particular, Laurie Hanna our patient number one, and then Saralee Berman, Mark's wife – gave us their trust, something for which there is no price.

ADDENDUM

History of Adipose Derived Stromal
Vascular Fraction Stem Cells

The following information was gleaned from numerous reports, papers and journals prepared by colleagues of the authors – Jackie See, MD and Dennis Ling. This is a chronological report of those findings.

2001
Zuk PhD, and her associates at the laboratory for regenerative bioengineering and repair, UCLA School of Medicine, Los Angeles, California, USA, determined that a population of stem cells could be isolated from human adipose tissue via processed lipoaspirate (PLA), suction-assisted lipectomy, better known as liposuction. These cells could be maintained in vitro for extended periods. PLA cells are of mesodermal or mesenchymal origin. These cells differentiate in vitro into adipogenic, chondrogenic, myogenic, and osteogenic cells in the presence of lineage-specific induction factors.

2002
Stafford, et al., examined whether murine and human adipose-derived adult stem (ADAS) cells can be induced to undergo neuronal differentiation. They isolated ADAS cells from the adipose tissue of adult BalbC mice or from human liposuction tissue and induced neuronal differentiation with valproic acid, butylated hydroxyanisole, insulin, and hydrocortisone. Again in 2002, Zuk, et al, Published another paper on their continuing research of isolating human adipose stem cells.

Zuk et al., Adipose tissue, like bone marrow, is derived from the mesenchyme and contains a stroma that is easily isolated. Preliminary studies have recently identified a putative stem cell population within the adipose stromal compartment.

2003
Cousin, et al, published findings on the Reconstitution of lethally irradiated mice by cells isolated from adipose tissue. They determined that adipose tissue can expand throughout adult life and its expansion is not only due to mature adipocyte hypertrophy but also to the presence of precursor cells in stroma-vascular fraction (SVF).

Ashjian, et al, also from the UCLA Medical Center for Regenerative Bioengineering, reported in their findings that PLA cells can be induced to differentiate into early neural progenitors, which are of an ectodermal origin. Once again in 2003, **Dragoo, et al,** Published in the Journal of Bone and Joint Surgery, that tissue-Tissue-engineered cartilage and bone using stem cells from human infrapatellar fat pads. They extracted multipotential processed lipoaspirate (PLA) cells from five human infrapatellar fat pads and embedded into fibrin glue nodules]

Dragoo et al., To date, differentiation to nonmesodermal fates has not been reported. This study demonstrates that PLA cells can be induced to differentiate into early neural progenitors, which are of an ectodermal origin]

2004
Bacou, et al, published their findings that transplantation of adipose tissue-derived stromal cells increases mass and functional capacity of damaged skeletal muscle. Adipose tissue stromal cells labeled with Adv cyto LacZ from 3-day-old primary cultures (SVF1) were autotransplanted into damaged tibialis anterior muscles. Fifteen days later, beta-galactosidase staining of regenerated fibers was detected, showing participation of these cells in muscle regeneration.

Cowan, et al, of Stanford University of Medicine, published their findings that adipose-derived adult stromal cells heal critical-size mouse calvarial defects. Their study investigated the in vivo osteogenic capability of adipose-derived adult stromal (ADAS) cells, BMS cells, calvarial-derived osteoblasts and dura mater cells to heal critical-size mouse calvarial defects.

Safford et al, Duke University Medical Center, published their research results on the characterization of neuronal/glial differentiation of murine adipose-derived adult stromal cells. They extended these observations to test the hypothesis that murine (mu) ADAS cells can be induced to exhibit characteristics of neuronal and glial tissue by exposure to a cocktail of induction agents. Still in 2004, **Guilak, et al**, also of the Duke University Medical Center, published a paper on '**Adipose-derived Adult Stem Cells for Cartilage Tissue engineering**'. They deemed that ADAS cells show significant promise for the development of functional tissue replacements for various tissues of the musculoskeletal system.

Miranville, A, et al., Department of Cardiovascular Physiology, J-W Goethe University, Frankfurt, Germany, published their findings on the Improvement of postnatal neovascularization by human adipose tissue-derived stem cells, to characterize the cell populations that compose the SVF of human AT originating from subcutaneous and visceral depots, fluorescence-activated cell sorter analysis was performed by use of fluorescent antibodies directed against the endothelial and stem cell markers CD31, CD34, CD133, and ABCG2.

Guilak, et al., ADAS cells show significant promise for the development of functional tissue replacements for various tissues of the musculoskeletal system.

Kang SK et al., of Tulane University Health Sciences Center, showed in their research on neurogenesis of rhesus adipose stromal cells, that they isolated and characterized a population **of non-human primate adipose tissue stromal** cells (pATSCs) containing multipotent progenitor cells. They showed that these pATSCs can differentiate into several mesodermal lineages, as well as neural lineage cells.

Lendeckel S, et al., Justus-Liebig-University Medical School, Giessen, Germany, published their findings on **autologous stem cells (adipose)**

and fibrin glue used to treat widespread traumatic calvarial defects. This was a report of **a 7-year-old girl** suffering from widespread calvarial defects after severe head injury with multifragment calvarial fractures, decompressive craniectomy for refractory intracranial hypertension and replantation of cryopreserved skull fragments. Postoperative course was uneventful and CT-scans showed new bone formation and near complete calvarial continuity three months after the reconstruction.

2005

Seo MJ, et al., of the Pusan National University, Pusan 602-739, Republic of Korea, reported their findings on the differentiation of human adipose stromal cells into hepatic lineage in vitro and in vivo. They found that mesenchymal stem cells isolated from human adipose tissue are immunocompatible and are easily isolated. Therefore, hADSC may become an alternative source to hepatocyte regeneration or liver cell transplantation. At the Department of Medicine/Nephrology, Johann Wolfgang Goethe-University, Frankfurt, Germany,

Brzoska M, et al., published findings on epithelial differentiation of human adipose tissue-derived adult stem cells. Their findings showed that ADAS-cells have epithelial potential. In 2005, from the UCLA Department of Urology,

Jack, et al., studied processed lipoaspirate cells for tissue engineering of the lower urinary tract and implications for the treatment of stress urinary incontinence and bladder reconstruction. PLA cells are an easily accessible source of pluripotent cells, them ideal fotr tissue regeneration. PLA cells may provide a feasible and cost-effective cell source for urinary tract reconstruction.

2006

Conejero JA, et al., Division of Plastic and Reconstructive Surgery, New York Presbyterian Hospital, studies the repair of palatal bone defects using osteogenically differentiated fat-derived stem cells. Their study demonstrated the feasibility of reconstructing bony defects with fat-derived stem cells. In Switzerland, at the Department of Research, University Hospital in Basal,

Timper, et al., found that human adipose tissue-derived mesenchymal stem cells differentiate into insulin, somatostatin, and glucagon expressing cells. Using quantitative PCR a down-regulation of ABCG2 and up-regulation of pancreatic developmental transcription factors Isl-1, Ipf-1, and Ngn3 were observed together with induction of the islet hormones insulin, glucagon, and somatostatin.

Rodriguez LV, et al., also from the UCLA Department of Urology, found that adipose-derived cells have the potential to differentiate into functional smooth muscle cells and, thus, adipose tissue can be a useful source of cells for treatment of injured tissues where smooth muscle plays an important role. Their findins showed that clonogenic multipotent stem cells in human adipose tissue differentiate into functional smooth muscle cells.

2007

Fang B, et al., from the Department of Hematology, Henan Institute of Hematology, 127 Dongming Road, hengzhou, Henan, China, reported in their findings that using human adipose tissue-derived mesenchymal stem cells as salvage therapy for hepatic graft-versus-host disease resembling acute hepatitis concluded that it is worthwhile to administer AMSC as a treatment for common hepatic GVHD, particularly for atypical cases presenting as acute hepatitis. A 43-year-old woman with chronic hepatic graft-versus-host disease (GVHD) who failed previous immunosuppressive therapy with cyclosporine and prednisone was treated with tacrolimus starting on day 165 after allogeneic hematopoietic stem cell transplantation.

Banas A, et al., at the National Cancer Center Research Institute, Tokyo, Japan, found recent observations indicate that several stem cells can differentiate into hepatocytes; thus, cell-based therapy is a potential alternative to liver transplantation. They used AT-MSCs from different age patients and found that, after incubation with specific growth factors (hepatocyte growth factor [HGF], fibroblast growth factor [FGF1], FGF4) the CD105(+) fraction of AT-MSCs exhibited high hepatic differentiation ability in an adherent monoculture condition.

Kim, et al., studied the systemic transplantation of human adipose stem cells attenuated cerebral inflammation and degeneration in a hemorrhagic stroke model. They reported that ASC's, adipose-derived stem cells, are readily accessible multipotent mesenchymal stem cells and are known to secrete multiple growth factors. They found that ASCs transplantation in the ICH model reduced both acute cerebral inflammation and chronic brain degeneration, and promoted long-term functional recovery.

Mauney JR, et al., Department of Biomedical Engineering, Tufts University, 4 Colby Street, Medford, MA 02155, USA., studied engineering adipose-like tissue in vitro and in vivo utilizing human bone marrow and adipose-derived mesenchymal stem cells with silk fibroin 3D scaffolds. Their results suggested that macro porous 3D AB and HEIP silk fibroin scaffolds offer an important platform for cell-based adipose tissue engineering applications.

Heydarkhan-Hagvall S, et al., at the Regenerative Bioengineering and Repair Laboratory, at UCLA, Los Angeles, Calif., USA., published their paper, **"Human adipose stem cells: a potential cell source for cardiovascular tissue engineering.** Their results indicate that hASCs are a potential cell source for cardiovascular tissue engineering; however, the differentiation capacity of hASCs into SMCs and ECs is passage number- and culture condition-dependent. As it was in 2004, 2008 was a very productive year for ADSC research. Hsu et al., at the University of Wisconsin, studied the efficacy of bone morphogenetic protein (BMP)-2-producing adipose-derived stem cells in inducing a posterolateral spine fusion in an athymic rat model. In one group of eight rats, spinal fusion was demonstrated to be successful.

Hsu, et al., Adipose-derived stem cells show promise as gene transduction targets for inducing bone formation to enhance spinal fusion in biologically stringent environments.

Park BS, et al., at the Division of Stem Cell Research, Prostemics Research Institute, Seoul, Korea, published their findings concerning adipose-derived stem cells. ADSCs and their secretory factors show promise for application in cosmetic dermatology, especially in the treatment of skin aging.

Trottier V, et al., Laboratoire d'Organogénèse Expérimentale Quebec, Canada, reported using human adipose-derived stem/stromal cells for the production of new skin substitutes. By exploiting the adipogenic potential of ASCs, they produced a more complete trilayered skin substitute consisting of the epidermis, the dermis, and the adipocyte-containing hypodermis, the skin's deepest layer.

Xu Y, et al., at the Department of Neurology, Zhejiang University, PR China, in studying the myelin-forming ability of Schwann cell-like cells induced from rat adipose-derived stem cells in vitro, determined that SC-like cells induced from adipose-derived stem cells (ADSC) may be one of the ideal alternative cell systems for SC. Their data demonstrated that SC-like cells from ADSC were able to form myelins and these cells may benefit the treatment of peripheral and central nerve injuries.

2009

Okura et al., published their findings on transdifferentiation of human adipose-derived stromal cells into insulin-producing clusters, in The Japanese Society for Artificial Organs Journal, 2009. They reported that the autoimmune destruction of insulin-producing beta cells is the cause of type 1 Diabetes mellitus. They feel that their insulin-producing cells derived from ADSCs could potentially be used for cell therapy of type 1 diabetes mellitus.

<u>Nakada A</u>, et al., at the Department of Bioartificial Organs, Institute for Frontier Medical Sciences, Kyoto University, Japan, published their findings on the regeneration of central nervous tissue using a collagen scaffold and adipose-derived stromal cells. Their data suggests that ASCs seeded into a collagen scaffold may have the potential to promote regeneration of nervous tissue after cerebral cortex injury.

Kondo et al., at the Department of Cardiology, Nagoya University Graduate School of Medicine, Nagoya, Japan, reported on their study of the implantation of adipose-derived regenerative cells enhancing ischemia-induced angiogenesis. They concluded Adipose tissue would be a valuable source for cell-based therapeutic angiogenesis. Moreover, chemokine SDF-1 may play a pivotal role in the ADRCs-mediated angiogenesis at least in part by facilitating mobilization of EPCs.

Garcia-Olmo D, et al., Department of Surgery and Cell Therapy, La Paz University Hospital, Madrid, Spain reported their findings on the administration of expanded ASCs (20 to 60 million cells) in combination with fibrin glue is an effective and safe treatment for complex perianal fistula and appears to achieve higher rates of healing than fibrin glue alone. Patients with complex perianal fistulas associated with Crohn's were randomly assigned to intralesional treatment with fibrin glue or fibrin glue plus 20 million ASCs. Fistula healing and quality of life were evaluated at eight weeks and one year. If healing was not seen at eight weeks, a second dose of fibrin glue or fibrin glue plus 40 million ASCs was administered. They reported that the administration of expanded ASCs (20 to 60 million cells) in combination with fibrin glue is an effective and safe treatment for complex perianal fistula and appears to achieve higher rates of healing than fibrin glue alone.

Lin et al., school of Medicine, Department of Urology, University of California-Knuppe Molecular Urology Laboratory, San Francisco, studied the potential of adipose-derived stem cells for treatment of erectile dysfunction. The adipose derived stem cells are paravascularly localized in the adipose tissue, and under specific induction medium conditions, these cells differentiated into neuron-like cells, smooth muscle cells and endothelium in vitro. The ADSCs are a potential source for stem cell-based therapies, which imply the possibility of an effective clinical therapy for ED in the near future.

Puissant et al., Laboratoire d'Immunologie, Toulouse France, reported their findings on the **Immunomodulatory effect of human adipose tissue-derived adult stem cells: comparison with bone marrow mesenchymal stem cells.** Like mesenchymal stem cells from bone marrow (BM-MSCs), adipose tissue-derived adult stem cells (ADAS cells) can differentiate into several lineages and present therapeutical potential for repairing damaged tissues.

Riordan et al., Medistem Inc, San Diego, CA, USA, published their findings in the Journal of Translational Medicine, on '**Non-expanded adipose stromal vascular fraction cell therapy for multiple sclerosis.'** In this paper, they discussed the rationale for use of autologous SVF in treatment of multiple sclerosis and described their experiences with three patients. Based on this rationale and initial experiences, we propose controlled trials of autologous SVF in various inflammatory conditions. They treated three patients with varying levels of MS. The patients treated were part of a compassionate-use evaluation of stem cell therapeutic protocols in a physician-initiated manner. Previous experiences in MS patients using allogeneic CD34+ cord blood cells together with MSC did not routinely result in substantial improvements observed in the three cases described above. While obviously no conclusions in terms of therapeutic efficacy can be drawn from the above reports, we believe that further clinical evaluation of autologous SVF cells is warranted in autoimmune conditions.

Gonzales et al., Tres Cantos, and Fundación Centro Nacional de Investigaciones Cardiovasculares Madrid, Spain, published in the Arthritis Care & Research Journal, the '**Treatment of experimental arthritis by inducing immune tolerance with human adipose-derived mesenchymal stem cells.**' Mice with collagen-induced arthritis were treated with human AD-MSCs after disease onset, and clinical scores were determined. Inflammatory response was determined by measuring the levels of different mediators of inflammation in the joints and serum. Systemic infusion of human AD-MSCs significantly reduced the incidence and severity of experimental arthritis. Human AD-MSCs emerge as key regulators of immune tolerance by inducing the generation/activation of Treg cells and are thus attractive candidates for a cell-based therapy for RA.

Froelich et al., Division of Cardiovascular Diseases, Mayo Clinic, Rochester, MN 55905, USA, reported in their findings that Adipose tissue is an abundant source of endothelial cells as well as stem and progenitor cells which can develop an endothelial phenotype. It has been demonstrated that these cells have distinct angiogenic properties in vitro and in vivo. These data suggest that ADECs represent an autologous source of proliferative endothelial cells, which demonstrate the capacity to rapidly improve reendothelialization, improve vascular reactivity, and decrease intimal formation in a carotid artery injury model.

Gonzalez-Reyetal., School of Medicine, University of Seville, Seville, Spain, reported in their paper on '**Human adult stem cells derived**

from adipose tissue protect against experimental colitis and sepsis', that acute and chronic colitis was induced in mice with dextran sulfate sodium, and sepsis was induced by caecal ligation and puncture or by endotoxin injection. Colitic and septic mice were treated intraperitoneally with hASCs or murine ASCs, and diverse disease clinical signs and mortality was determined. Their conclusion was hASCs emerge as key regulators of immune/inflammatory responses in vivo and as attractive candidates for cell-based treatments for IBD and sepsis.

Lee et al., at the Department of Neurology, Clinical Research Institute, Seoul National University Hospital, Seoul, South Korea, slowed progression in models of Huntington disease by adipose stem cell transplantation. In a quinolinic acid (QA)-induced rat model of striatal degeneration, human ASCs (1 million cells) were transplanted into the ipsilateral striatal border immediately after the QA injection. human ASCs reduced apomorphine-induced rotation behavior, lesion volume, and striatal apoptosis. Adipose-derived stem cells (ASCs) are readily accessible and secrete multiple growth factors. Here, we show that ASC transplantation rescues the striatal pathology of Huntington disease (HD) models.

Ryu HH, et al., published their findings on **Functional recovery and neural differentiation after transplantation of allogenic adipose-derived stem cells in a canine model of acute spinal cord injury,** in the Journal of Veterinary Science. In their study, they evaluated if the implantation of allogenic adipose-derived stem cells (ASCs) improved neurological function in a canine spinal cord injury model. Results suggest that improvements of neurological function after transplantation of ASCs to dogs with spinal cord injuries might be partially due to neural differentiation of implanted stem cells.

Lin G, et al., at the University of California, San Francisco, California, USA, reported the derivation of insulin-producing cells from human or rat ADSC by transduction with the pancreatic duodenal homeobox 1 (Pdx1) gene. RT-PCR analyses showed that native ADSC expressed insulin, glucagon, and NeuroD genes that were up-regulated following Pdx1 transduction. ELISA analyses showed that the transduced cells secreted increasing amount of insulin in response to increasing concentration of glucose.

2010

Kajiyama et al., published their findings in The International Journal of Developmental Biology, that the human Pdx1 gene was transduced and expressed in murine adipose tissue-derived stem cells (ASCs). To evaluate pancreatic repair, they used a **mouse model** of pancreatic damage resulting in hyperglycemia, which involves injection of mice with streptozotocin (STZ). **STZ-treated mice** transplanted with Pdx1-transduced ASCs. The ease and safety associated with extirpating high numbers of cells from adipose tissues support the applicability of this system to developing a new cell therapy for IDDM. Results suggested that dx1-ASCs are stably engrafted in the pancreas and that high numbers of cells from adipose tissue support the development of a new cell therapy for IDDM.

Long et al., published their in The American Larygological, Rhinological and Octological Society, on the potential treatment option for severe vocal fold scarring is to replace the vocal fold cover layer with a tissue-engineered structure containing autologous cells. As a first step toward that goal, we sought to develop a three-dimensional cell-populated matrix resembling the vocal fold layers of lamina propria and epithelium. A three-dimensional structure of fibrin and adipose-derived stem cells was created as a prototype vocal fold replacement. Two segregated cell phenotypes occurred, producing a bilayered structure resembling epithelium over lamina propria. This preliminary work demonstrates the feasibility of tissue engineering to produce structures for vocal fold replacement.

Gonzalez-Rey et al., at the School of Medicine, University of Seville, Seville, Spain, found that human adipose-derived mesenchymal stem cells reduce inflammatory and T cell responses and induce regulatory T cells in vitro in rheumatoid arthritis. Adult mesenchymal stem cells were recently found to suppress effector T cell and inflammatory responses and have emerged as attractive therapeutic candidates for immune disorders. In rheumatoid arthritis (RA), a loss in the immunological self-tolerance causes the activation of autoreactive T cells against joint components and subsequent chronic inflammation. In conclusion, their work identified hASCs as key regulators of immune tolerance, with the capacity to suppress T cell and inflammatory responses and to induce the generation/activation of antigen-specific regulatory T cells.

Josiah et al., Brain Tumor Center of Excellence, Department of Neurosurgery, Wake Forest University School of Medicine, Winston-Salem, North Carolina, published their findings on **Adipose-derived stem cells as therapeutic delivery vehicles of an oncolytic virus for Glioblastoma,** in Molecular Therapy, the official journal of the American Society for Gene & Cell Therapy. They found that glioblastoma multiforme (GBM) accounts for the majority of primary malignant brain tumors and remains virtually incurable despite extensive surgical resection, radiotherapy, and chemotherapy. They hypothesized that adipose-derived stem cells (ADSCs) possess the ability to home and deliver myxoma virus to glioma cells and experimental gliomas. They infected ADSCs with vMyxgfp and found them to be permissive for myxoma virus replication. Their data suggests that ADSCs are promising new carriers of oncolytic viruses, specifically myxoma virus, to brain tumors.

Okura et al., Department of Somatic Stem Cell Therapy, Foundation for Biomedical Research and Innovation, Kobe, Japan, published their findings on **Cardiomyoblast-like cells differentiated from human adipose tissue-derived mesenchymal stem cells improve left ventricular dysfunction and survival in a rat myocardial infarction model.** They examined whether human ADMSCs (hADMSCs) could differentiate into cardiomyoblast-like cells (CLCs) by induction with dimethylsulfoxide and whether the cells would be utilized to treat cardiac dysfunction. Dimethylsulfoxide induced the expression of various cardiac markers in hADMSCs, such as alpha-cardiac actin, cardiac myosin light chain, and myosin heavy chain; none of which were detected in noncommitted hADMSCs. The induced cells were thus designated as hADMSC-derived CLCs (hCLCs). To confirm their beneficial effect on cardiac function, hCLC patches were transplanted onto the Nude rat myocardial infarction model, and compared with noncommitted hADMSC patch transplants and sham operations. Echocardiography demonstrated significant short-term improvement of cardiac function in both the patch-transplanted groups. However, long-term follow-up showed rescue and maintenance of cardiac function in the hCLC patch-transplanted group only, but not in the noncommitted hADMSC patch-transplanted animals. The hCLCs, but not the hADMSCs, engrafted into the scarred myocardium and differentiated into human cardiac troponin I-positive cells, and thus regarded as cardiomyocytes. Transplantation of the hCLC patches also resulted in recovery of cardiac function and improvement of long-term survival rate.

Uysal AC, et al., studied tendon regeneration and repair with adipose derived stem cells, at the Department of Plastic and Reconstructive Surgery, Baskent University, Faculty of Medicine, Bahcelievler, Ankara, Turkey. Tendon, the crucial element of the musculoskeletal system, when damaged, never restores the biological and biomechanical properties completely. ASCs present an ideal cell source for experimental and clinical research on tendon engineering.

Li K, et al., at the Institute of Basic Medical Sciences and School of Basic Medicine, People's Republic of China, investigated the differentiation characteristics and the role of MSCs in renal tubular injury, human adipose-derived MSCs (hAD-MSCs) were transplanted into ischemia-reperfusion (I/R) kidneys in C57BL/6 mouse model. Results showed that hAD-MSCs were able to differentiate toward renal tubular epithelium at an early stage of injuries. The differentiated donor cells replaced the vacant space left over by the dead cells, contributed to maintenance of structural integrity and preceded to a subsequent tissue repair process. Furthermore, MSCs as supportive cells may promote repair via secreting cytokines. The differentiation and replacement of MSCs at an extremely early stage play important roles for the subsequent self-repair and -renewal of functional cells. Direct differentiation of MSCs, as an important mechanism of injured kidney repair, warrants further investigation.

di Summa et al., Chirurgie Plastique et Reconstructive CHUV, Université de Lausanne, Rue de Bugnon 46, 1005 Lausanne, CH, Switzerland, decided to test new fibrin nerve conduits seeded with various cell types (primary Schwann cells and adult stem cells differentiated to a Schwann cell-like phenotype) for repair of sciatic nerve injury. Two weeks after implantation, the conduits were removed and examined by immunohistochemistry for axonal regeneration (evaluated by PGP 9.5 expression) and Schwann cell presence (detected by S100 expression).

The results show a significant increase in axonal regeneration in the group of fibrin seeded with Schwann cells compared with the empty fibrin conduit. They published their findings in an International Journal of Surgical Reconstruction.

REFERENCES

1. Zuk et al., Multilineage cells from human adipose tissue: implications for cell-based therapies. Tissue Eng. 2001;7:211–228. [PubMed]
2. Safford et al., Neurogenic differentiation of murine and human adipose-derived stromal cells. Biochem. Biophys. Res. Commun. 2002;294:371–379. [PubMed]
3. Zuk et al., Human adipose tissue is a source of multipotent stem cells. Mol. Biol. Cell. 2002;13:4279–4295. [PMC free article] [PubMed]
4. Cousin et al., Reconstitution of lethally irradiated mice by cells isolated from adipose tissue. Biochem. Biophys. Res. Commun. 2003;21:1016–1022. [PubMed]
5. Ashjian et al., In vitro differentiation of human processed lipoaspirate cells into early neural progenitors. Plast. Reconstr. Surg. 2003;111:1922–1931. [PubMed]
6. Dragoo et al., Tissue-engineered cartilage and bone using stem cells from human infrapatellar fat pads. J. Bone Joint Surg. Br. 2003;85:740–747. [PubMed]
7. Bacou et al., Transplantation of adipose tissue-derived stromal cells increases mass and functional capacity of damaged skeletal muscle. Cell Transplant. 2004;13:103–111. [PubMed]
8. Cowan et al., Adipose-derived adult stromal cells heal critical-size mouse calvarial defects. Nat. Biotechnol. 2004;22:560–567. [PubMed]
9. Safford et al., Characterization of neuronal/glial differentiation of murine adipose-derived adult stromal cells. Exp. Neurol. 2004;187:319–328. [PubMed]

10. Guilak et al., Adipose-derived adult stem cells for cartilage tissue engineering. Biorheology. 2004;41:389–399. [PubMed]

11. Miranville et al., Improvement of postnatal neovascularization by human adipose tissue-derived stem cells. Circulation. 2004;110:349–355. [PubMed]

12. Kang et al., Neurogenesis of Rhesus adipose stromal cells. J. Cell Sci. 2004;117:4289–4299. [PubMed]

13. Lendeckel et al., Autologous stem cells (adipose) and fibrin glue used to treat widespread traumatic calvarial defects: case report. J. Craniomaxillofac. Surg. 2004;32:370–373. [PubMed]

14. Seo et al., Differentiation of human adipose stromal cells into hepatic lineage in vitro and in vivo. Biochem. Biophys. Res. Commun. 2005;328:258–264. [PubMed]

15. Brzoska et al., Epithelial differentiation of human adipose tissue-derived adult stem cells. Biochem. Biophys. Res. Commun. 2005;330:142–150. [PubMed]

16. Jack et al., Processed lipoaspirate cells for tissue engineering of the lower urinary tract: implications for the treatment of stress urinary incontinence and bladder reconstruction. J. Urol. 2005;174:2041–2045. [PubMed]

17. Conejero et al., Repair of palatal bone defects using osteogenically differentiated fat-derived stem cells. Plast. Reconstr. Surg. 2006;117:857–863. [PubMed]

18. Timper et al., Human adipose tissue-derived mesenchymal stem cells differentiate into insulin, somatostatin, and glucagon expressing cells. Biochem. Biophys. Res. Commun. 2006;341:1135–1140. [PubMed]

19. Rodriguez et al., Clonogenic multipotent stem cells in human adipose tissue differentiate into functional smooth muscle cells. Proc. Natl. Acad. Sci. USA. 2006;103:12167–12172. [PMC free article] [PubMed]

20. Fang et al., Using human adipose tissue-derived mesenchymal stem cells as salvage therapy for hepatic graft-versus-host disease resembling acute hepatitis. Transplant. Proc. 2007;39:1710–1713. [PubMed]

21. Banas et al., Adipose tissue-derived mesenchymal stem cells as a source of human hepatocytes. Hepatology. 2007;46:219–228. [PubMed]

22. Kim et al,. Systemic transplantation of human adipose stem cells attenuated cerebral inflammation and degeneration in a hemorrhagic stroke model. Brain Res. 2007;1183:43–50. [PubMed]

23. Mauney et al., Engineering adipose-like tissue in vitro and in vivo utilizing human bone marrow and adipose-derived mesenchymal stem cells with silk fibroin 3D scaffolds. Biomaterials. 2007;28:5280–5290. [PMC free article] [PubMed]

24. Heydarkhan-Hagvall et al., Human adipose stem cells: a potential cell source for cardiovascular tissue engineering. Cells Tissues Organs. 2008;187:263–274. [PubMed]

25. Hsu W. et al., Stem cells from human fat as cellular delivery vehicles in an athymic rat posterolateral spine fusion model. J Bone Joint Surg. Am. 2008;90:1043–1052. [PubMed]

26. Park et al., Adipose-derived stem cells and their secretory factors as a promising therapy for skin aging. Dermatol. Surg. 2008;34:1323–1326. [PubMed]

27. Trottier et al., IFATS collection: using human adipose-derived stem/stromal cells for the production of new skin substitutes. Stem Cells. 2008;26:2713–2723. [PubMed]

28. Xu et al., Myelin-forming ability of Schwann cell-like cells induced from rat adipose-derived stem cells in vitro. Brain Res. 2008;1239:49–55. [PubMed]

29. Okura et al., Transdifferentiation of human adipose tissue-derived stromal cells into insulin-producing clusters. J. Artif. Organs. 2009a;12:123–130. [PubMed]

30. Nakada et al., Regeneration of central nervous tissue using a collagen scaffold and adipose-derived stromal cells. Cells Tissues Organs. 2009;190:326–335. [PubMed]

31. Kondo et al., Implantation of adipose-derived regenerative cells enhances ischemia-induced angiogenesis. Arterioscler. Thromb. Vasc. Biol. 2009;29:61–66. [PubMed]

32. Garcia-Olmo et al., Expanded adipose-derived stem cells for the treatment of complex perianal fistula: a phase II clinical trial. Dis. Colon Rectum. 2009;52:79–86. [PubMed]

33. Lin et al., Potential of adipose-derived stem cells for treatment of erectile dysfunction. J Sex Med. 2009a;6(Suppl 3):320–327. [PMC free article] [PubMed]

34. Puissant et al., Immunomodulatory effect of human adipose tissue-derived adult stem cells: comparison with bone marrow mesenchymal stem cells. Br. J. Haematol. 2005;129:118–129. [PubMed]

35. Riordan et al., Non-expanded adipose stromal vascular fraction cell therapy for multiple sclerosis. J. Transl. Med. 2009;7:29. [PMC free article] [PubMed]

36. Gonzalez et al., Treatment of experimental arthritis by inducing immune tolerance with human adipose-derived mesenchymal stem cells. Arthritis Rheum. 2009;60:1006–1019. [PubMed]

37. Froehlich et al., Carotid repair using autologous adipose-derived endothelial cells. Stroke. 2009;40:1886–1891. [PMC free article] [PubMed]

38. Gonzalez-Rey et al., Human adult stem cells derived from adipose tissue protect against experimental colitis and sepsis. Gut. 2009;58:929–939. [PubMed]

39. Lee et al., Slowed progression in models of Huntington disease by adipose stem cell transplantation. Ann. Neurol. 2009;66:671–681. [PubMed]

40. Ryu et al., Functional recovery and neural differentiation after transplantation of allogenic adipose-derived stem cells in a canine model of acute spinal cord injury. J. Vet. Sci. 2009;10:273–284. [PMC free article] [PubMed]

41. Lin et al., Treatment of type 1 diabetes with adipose tissue-derived stem cells expressing pancreatic duodenal homeobox 1. Stem Cells Dev. 2009b;18:1399–1406. [PMC free article] [PubMed]

42. Kajiyama et al., Pdx1-transfected adipose tissue-derived stem cells differentiate into insulin-producing cells in vivo and reduce hyperglycemia in diabetic mice. Int. J. Dev. Biol. 2010;54:699–705. [PubMed]

43. Long et al., Epithelial differentiation of adipose-derived stem cells for laryngeal tissue engineering. Laryngoscope. 2009;120:125–131. [PubMed]

44. Gonzalez-Rey et al., Human adipose-derived mesenchymal stem cells reduce inflammatory and T cell responses and induce regulatory T cells in vitro in rheumatoid arthritis. [PubMed]

45. Josiah et al., Adipose-derived stem cells as therapeutic delivery vehicles of an oncolytic virus for glioblastoma. Mol. Ther. 2010;18:377–385. [PMC free article] [PubMed]

46. Okura et al., Cardiomyoblast-like cells differentiated from human adipose tissue-derived mesenchymal stem cells improve left ventricular dysfunction and survival in a rat myocardial infarction model. Tissue Eng. 2009c Part C Methods *Epub ahead of print.* [PubMed]

47. Uysal et al., Tendon regeneration and repair with adipose derived stem cells. Curr. Stem Cell Res. Ther. 2009 *Epub ahead of print.* [PubMed]

48. Li et al., Not a process of simple vicariousness, the differentiation of human adipose-derived mesenchymal stem cells to renal tubular epithelial cells plays an important role in acute kidney injury repairing. Stem Cells Dev. 2009 *Epub ahead of print.* [PubMed]

49. di Summa et al., Adipose-derived stem cells enhance peripheral nerve regeneration. J. Plast. Reconstr. Aesthet. Surg. 2009 *Epub ahead of print.* [PubMed]

Made in the USA
San Bernardino, CA
24 July 2016